Neurofeedback

Transforming Your Life
With Brain Biofeedback

Dr. Clare Albright
Clinical Psychologist

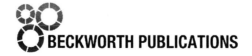

BECKWORTH PUBLICATIONS

Published by Beckworth Publications
3108 E. 10th St
Trenton, Mo 64683
www.BeckworthPublications.com

ISBN   978-0-9818791-5-4
Library of Congress Catalog Card Number: 2010900870

Terms of Use Agreement
This is a legally binding agreement between
readers and Beckworth Publications

Praise For

"Neurofeedback"

Transforming Your Life with Brain Biofeedback"

"The best beginner's guide to neurofeedback that I have read."

Michael Landgraf
Publisher - AVS Journal

"I love this book.

Dr. Clare has such a refreshing and engaging way of explaining the amazing healing power of neurofeedback.

'Neurofeedback' will be a great introduction to potential clients and those who love and care about them.

It can be so difficult to explain neurofeedback and it's potential value to people – which is what makes this book an important and needed work."

~Woody Deryckx

"Dr. Clare 'knocked it out of the ballpark' with information presented in a manner that is informative, easy to understand and written with hope for many.

~ Dr. Patti Williams, Ph.D.
Professor of Psychology

If you have ever wanted to explore alternative therapies for anxiety, depression, ADD, migraines, chronic pain, addiction, and a myriad of other issues, then this is a book for you.

Dr. Clare Albright explains in an easily understood way, the benefits of this exciting treatment called "Neurofeedback."

~ Ruth Butler, Marriage and Family Therapist

In *Neurofeedback: Transforming Your Life with Brain Biofeedback,* Dr. Clare has done a fantastic job of explaining the process, the benefits, and the background of neurofeedback.

Whether you are a clinician, a student, or just curious about neurofeedback, you will find this book to be both informative and refreshing. Dr. Clare explains this groundbreaking therapy in a way that everyone can understand.

I highly recommend this book to anyone who wants to learn more about neurofeedback and the successes that people have had with it.

~ Kelly Marquize

I was truly excited after reading Dr. Albright's book, "Neurofeedback" on neurofeedback because I felt that now so many more people will be able to get an understanding about this treatment form.

She writes in a way that anyone can understand what neurofeedback is, and how it can be such a beneficial treatment option for many conditions involving the brain.

If you or anyone you know is suffering from a brain related disorder and are looking for a treatment that may be less harmful and even more effective than traditional treatments, this book is a must read.

It's always important to fully investigate your options for treatment, and in this book you can easily learn about methods that many professionals know little about.

~ John Halderman
http://effectivepersonaldevelopmentblog.com

Dr. Clare Albright does an amazing job at taking a complex subject and making it readable for the beginner!

~ Dr. Anne Swanson-Leadbetter
Professor, Argosy University Psychology Doctoral Program

"This book opens up a whole new intellectual spectrum - for *all* readers. I am delighted by the insight I could so easily absorb!"

~ Mellisa Stoker
http://www.youtube.com/mellisamouse

"Dr. Albright has provided for us all a sparkling introduction to the dimly understood field of neurofeedback.

Her warm and personable style makes this book not only highly readable, but highly enjoyable."

Dr. Laird Bridgman, Psy.D.
Fellow, Academy of Cognitive Therapy
www.bridgmandocs.com

With a passion for finding a helping others achieve total health, Dr. Albright combines years of research with her intense love for helping people overcome the labels they have been assigned.

Her caring devotion resonates throughout the book.

~ Kimberly Armstrong, M.A.
Marketing Communications Consultant

"This is an amazing introductory book,

particularly for the "lay-person"

who is looking to gain education and insight,

without being overwhelmed by in-depth knowledge

or needing to understand the scientific language

regarding neurofeedback.

Bravo!"

~ Dr. Cay Crosby, Psy.D.
Center for Discovery - Eating Disorders

"As a neurofeedback provider I am always looking for information and materials for my clients.

Dr. Clare's book is a jewel.

It cuts to the heart of neurofeedback and explains difficult concepts in a way that is understandable to my clients.

Thanks so much for a wonderful addition to the neurofeedback library."

www.TidewaterNeurofeedback.com

~ Mary Price, M.Ed, LPC

I love it Dr. Clare... you did exactly what you said you would do - and gave a "lay- person" a chance to understand.... kudos....it is well written!!!

I'm going to buy a copy of "Neurofeedback" for someone very close to me and others that I know who need to read this.

I am not a great reader and I just read the entire book in one sitting.

Kudos - and let's get this book out there!!!!

Sincerely and excitingly,

~ Stuart Dangar

"Simple, clear, and coherent!

This is one book you'll appreciate having."

~Sam Saleh
www.samswriting.com

DEDICATION

To my son Daniel:
My favorite thing about you is how good hearted you are -
and you're lots of fun.

Table of Contents

Foreword

Dr. Clare Albright has accomplished something impressive with this book. She has taken a subject that can sometimes be rather complex, and distilled it into an easy, and more importantly, enjoyable book to read.

Dr. Albright did not set out to dazzle us with her brilliance and her ability to use words that the average person finds impressive, yet confusing. No, instead, what shines brighter than the sun at high noon, is her ability to package the foundational concepts of neurofeedback, into short stories, anecdotes and humorous examples that flood our minds with colorful, lively pictures that leave us with that *"oh, now I get it!"* feeling. For this reason, Dr. Albright has paradoxically demonstrated her brilliance.

I'm proud to say I personally know Dr. Clare Albright. She has a heart as big as Texas, and is always asking *"What more can I do to make the world a better place?"* As you read her lovely book, you too, will feel her warmth radiating from the pages.

When I read a book, of course, I like to be educated about certain things, but to the degree that I am also being entertained, I know, or not, that my investment has been a good one. With that being said, my experience with this book was like owning stock that has just had a record setting year in profits.

Now, it's time to issue a warning: This book is not the pinnacle of exacting numbers, statistics and endless details, described with hard to pronounce and medically correct terms, when it comes to neurofeedback. Those books have been written, and, after priming your mind with this one, I can assure you, the information in those books will more easily find a slot in your mind to slide into; even, and, perhaps, especially, if you are already accustomed to more technical reading. The power of stories and metaphors to effectively convey information is astonishing-and proven.

Because you are reading this book, it's likely that you simply want to know how neurofeedback can help you, or someone else in your life. After you've read it, you'll find that it's done that and more.

Dr. Albright, I have no doubt that this book will serve as the catalyst that is responsible for men, women and children, worldwide, having their lives transformed by the intelligent application of this continually emerging tool of neurofeedback. Your efforts have already made a difference...thank you!

~Vincent Harris,
author of "The Productivity Epiphany",
www.VinceHarris.com

Introduction

When I decided to write this book, I had one specific audience in mind; people with no background in medicine, psychology or other related fields, who had never heard of neurofeedback, or had, but only in passing, and were simply curious about what neurofeedback is and how it might benefit them.

It has been said that when we desire to easily and effectively teach adults about something - when a book will serve as the vehicle - we should use words and descriptions that would make sense to someone in the 6th grade. I know there have been many late nights on Christmas Eve when I would have loved to have had the instructions written this way for putting my child's gifts together.

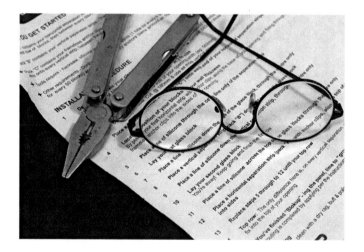

Brilliant people are often thought of as "brilliant" because of their ability to communicate clearly, and in simple language. Far too often what many think of as an offering of their brilliance, is little more than someone attempting to impress. All too often the only person who is impressed is the person who is speaking

Clearly, not everything we desire to know about is written or structured in this manner. Fortunately, this book is.

If you don't know your pre-frontal cortex from your medulla oblongata, and simply want a fun and easily understood description of neurofeedback and what it can do for you, then this book was the right choice.

Now, let me make one thing clear. There are several very good books about neurofeedback out there. And, after having read this book, any of them will be far more easily understood and absorbed if you choose to further your knowledge of neurofeedback and take it to a more technical level.

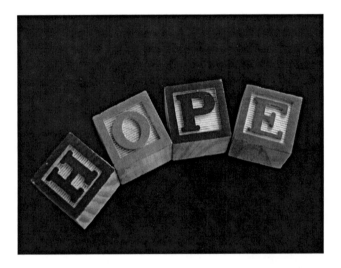

Have fun and relax, allowing your mind to embrace the metaphors and descriptions offered, feeling free to construct your own along the way; you may find my descriptions are just the catalyst for those you will create, and that ultimately, make even more sense to you.

Chapter 1

What are People Saying About Neurofeedback?

"All truth passes through three stages:
First it is ridiculed.
Second, it is violently opposed.
Third, it is accepted as being self-evident."

–Schopenhauer

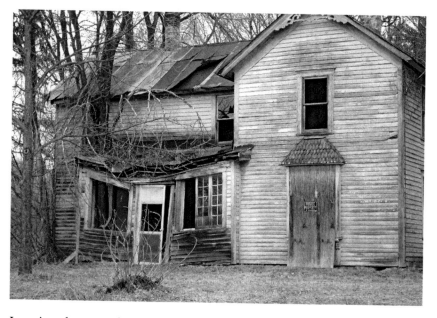

Imagine that one day, while you are out driving through a part of town you've never been to before, that you see man placing two large objects out in the front yard of an old run down house.

Curious, you pull over to watch and see what he's up to. Having noticed that you are watching, he motions for you to come join him. As you walk into the yard, he explains that he has just purchased the house, and is about to have the house fix and repair itself. In front of him, there is a large picture and a big full-length mirror.

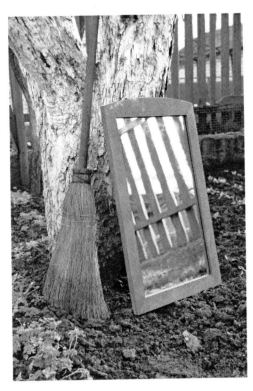

He tells you, *"Okay, I'm going to hold up the mirror so the house can see how it looks now, in its run down condition. At the same time, I'm going to hold up a picture that shows how the house once looked, just a few months after it was built, and still in tip top condition. By being able to see the changes as it is repairing itself, and, simultaneously having clear picture of what it will look like when it's done, the house can make all of the needed changes, all by itself!"*

Would you like to be able to have your home repair itself, naturally transforming and coming back to tip top shape? Me too. Unfortunately, a house can't do that. However, *the human brain can.*

Before I go much further, I'd like to address a couple of questions that many people like you might have after having just read a statement like "*The human brain can repair itself.*"

Here are the questions:

If this is true, and this neurofeedback stuff can get my brain to repair itself, why haven't I heard about it?

Why hasn't it been all over the news and in magazines?

Those are both great questions, and, I have a couple of really good answers.

First, neurofeedback has been written about by most of the top publications, and featured on many of the most popular television news shows. Time Magazine, ABC News, CBS, NBC, Fox News, Scientific American, and Psychology Today, just to name a few. They have all written or talked about the virtues of neurofeedback.

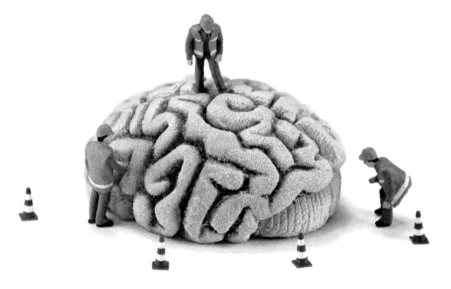

The main reason, I believe, that many people have not heard about neurofeedback, is that it simply gets lost in the shuffle of the almost unlimited number of sensationalized stories. Like it, or not, "feel good" stories don't sell nearly as well as the tragic ones. So, it's easy to only notice and remember the stories that evoke fear, and then miss many of the stories like those that look at a case study of someone who has been helped by neurofeedback, for example.

The second reason someone might have not yet heard about neurofeedback, is that, as I write, neurofeedback is not yet being taught in most medical schools or psychology programs.

Many people find it surprising to learn that only in recent years have medical students been required to take classes about nutrition. I think you'll agree: it's not that good nutrition wasn't important before they started being required to learn more about it in medical school, but it's just a simple matter of it not being a primary concern of most physicians before that time. As a result, you didn't hear nearly as much about it.

Neurofeedback Tip

Even as I write, the wave of excitement about the seemingly unlimited benefits of neurofeedback is rolling faster, and building more momentum with each passing day.

I don't remember any mention of neurofeedback, or EEG biofeedback as it is also called, from my time in graduate school. In many professions the latest improvements are learned by those newest to the field. In order for me to learn how to provide neurofeedback, I had to take time off work to attend continuing education classes. Then, I had to hire mentors, and pay them an hourly rate, to supervise me when first used the neurofeedback machine.

The costs of taking time off of work, attending days of continuing education, hiring supervisors, and purchasing expensive equipment and software is one of the reasons that neurofeedback has not become more well known.

Neurofeedback Tip

Neurofeedback can often be stopped after 30-40 sessions, with the patient remaining symptom free for decades.

Even as I write, the wave of excitement about the seemingly unlimited benefits of neurofeedback is rolling faster, and building more momentum with each passing day. The "masses" will have the opportunity to benefit only after neurofeedback becomes a household name. You don't have to wait, though. By the time you have finished reading this book, you will have a better understanding of neurofeedback, how it works, and what it can be used for, than almost anyone else around you.

Neurofeedback is not a cure-all; while you will find there to be a very diverse number of conditions for which neurofeedback *can* assist you in producing what can seem like, at times, miraculous results, there are also a large number of challenges for which neurofeedback would be of little help.

I'd also like to point out, that at the current time, there are still conditions that medication is still the most effective treatment available.

With that being said, the current research on neurofeedback shows that unlike treatment with a pharmaceutical intervention, where the medication will have to be taken for long periods of time - perhaps for a lifetime-to be free from the symptoms or challenges of a particular condition, neurofeedback can often be stopped after 30-40 sessions, with the patient remaining symptom free for decades. For some people, this alone makes neurofeedback a very compelling consideration.

I decided to write this book because I wanted to make the exciting possibilities of neurofeedback known to more people. I wanted to write a book that explained neurofeedback in terms that people could understand. I decided to use 'word pictures' to explain some of the complicated concepts surrounding EEG neurofeedback.

Chapter 2

The Fly is on the W[...]
Observing a Neurof[...]

Neurofeedback: Tr[...]

"Here in the ne[...]
tentiveness call[...]

The C[...]
Boy' [...]
in[...]

8

"All human evil comes from a single cause,
man's inability to sit still in a room."

–Blaise Pascal

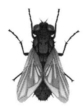

John Doe is a 36 year old man who has been referred to Dr. Albright for neurofeedback sessions. He enjoys his job as an engineer in the aerospace industry. "I've had trouble focusing all of my life, Dr. Albright. I am amazed that I've had this much success while having ADD. I've struggled with Attention Deficit Disorder since I started the first grade."

John has already been diagnosed with ADD by another psychologist, who gave him a full battery of tests, which included checklists that both John and his wife filled out. Both of them checked off words to describe John from the list such as 'distractible', 'impulsive', 'short attention span', and 'restless'.

Dr. Albright sits down in her comfortable, maroon leather office chair and begins to interview John, discussing the final report on John's testing that she received from the other psychologist. Dr. Albright's office looks like any other counseling office except for the small, grey neurofeedback machine on the desk. The neurofeedback machine's dimensions are 6" x 6", and 2" thick.

ofeedback office we administer a 15 minute test of at-
a 'Continuous Performance Test', or 'CPT' for short."

T, is a small white device that looks a lot like a small 'Game
ideo game. John holds the device for about 15 minutes and is
structed to click the device whenever an 'X' appears. This is John's
baseline score for attention versus inattention.

One of the tests that John brought with him to Dr. Albright's office is
his QEEG (Quantitative EEG) Brain Map. This map shows Dr. Albright
which parts of John's brain have abnormally low brainwave activity and
which parts have abnormally high brain wave activity.

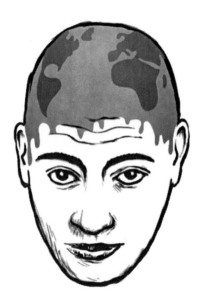

Based on the QEEG brain map results, Dr. Albright knows where to
place the leads on John's scalp for the first session. The QEEG brain
map report looks like a picture of 19 heads drawn on a piece of paper
with different colors on each of the heads to signify the level of brainwave activity. Each 'head' drawn in the report represents a different part
of John's scalp where a brainwave reading was taken.

It takes 5 minutes for Dr. Albright to get the leads in place on John's
scalp.

First Dr. Albright shows John a 'Pac Man' type of neurofeedback game on her computer screen. She begins to explain:

"In order to help your brainwaves to get to the normal range, there is going to be a reward signal from the computer whenever your brainwave activity moves closer to the normal range. The software signals your brain that it is moving towards the normal range with these reward tone sounds and with these games.

One of the rewards is that this 'Pac Man' will move around the Pac Man game board and 'eat the dots'. If your brainwaves don't move closer to the normal range, then the Pac Man will stay motionless and it won't be 'eating the dots'."

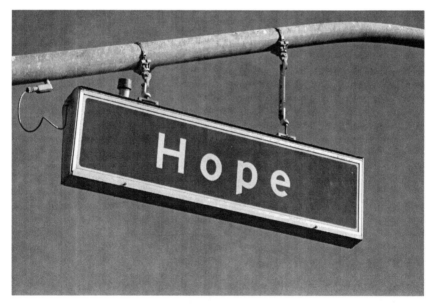

John begins to laugh as he watches the Pac Man move around the game board gobbling up the dots.

Dr. Albright continues, "I have the neurofeedback machine set up to be training several different brainwave patterns at once. Since you have an ADD diagnosis, we are encouraging the brainwaves that are used in focusing, which are called 'Beta' waves, by setting up the Pac Man to move when your Beta waves are increasing in frequency. We also set up the Pac Man to move when your relaxed brainwaves, or the 'Alpha' brainwaves, decrease in frequency."

Dr. Albright begins to show John several different games in her neurofeedback software collection. In one game, John notices that a spaceship flies through space whenever his brainwaves move closer to the normal range. In another game his brainwaves are rewarded by filling a jar with marbles when his brainwaves respond in the right direction. In a fourth game his brain is rewarded by a photo of a Golden Retriever becoming more visible each time his brainwaves move in the right direction.

The last part of the neurofeedback software that Dr. Albright shows John is a DVD player. She explains to John that "when your brainwaves move in the right direction the movie will appear on the screen and start playing. When your brainwaves are not responding in the right direction the movie will slow down and stop and the screen will fade out."

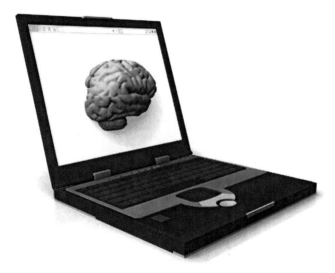

Dr. Albright shows John that the DVD inside of the player was one of the movies that John had brought with him to the session entitled 'The Bourne Identity'.

John starts laughing as he watches the beginning of the movie. He says "my brain is controlling my favorite movie. This is very motivating, Doc. How can I try harder so I get to see the whole movie?"

Dr. Albright chuckles and replies, "The amazing thing about neurofeedback is that your brain is doing all of the work. All you need to do is to allow yourself to observe the screen."

"That makes no sense, Doc. Isn't there any way that I can help this along? I'm a motivated client," John replied.

"It helps if you eat a healthy diet and get enough sleep. During the neurofeedback sessions your brain will actually be doing the work all on its own," Dr. Albright answers.

Neurofeedback Tip

During the neurofeedback sessions your brain will actually be doing the work all on its own.

John starts to scrunch up his face and his fists are clenched. The movie screen turns black and the movie soundtrack stops playing.

"O.K. Doc, I can see you're right. All of this effort is causing the opposite of what I want to happen with this movie."

At the end of the session Dr. Albright explains, "As your brain produces more and more of the correct type of brainwaves, I will re-adjust the settings on the neurofeedback software. It is similar to what an instructor does in the weight room when he wants to train an athlete to use bigger weights. The athlete may have started out only able to lift 150 lbs. with his legs, but by the end of training he may be able to lift 250 lbs. with his legs.

In the same way, I will be continually raising the settings on the neurofeedback machine as you attend more and more 'workout' sessions for your brain. Yes, some people do call neurofeedback brainwave sessions 'exercise'.

After enough sessions have passed, I will re-administer a simple version of the QEEG brain map test. I believe that your brain map will then show a normal amount of brainwave activity throughout your brain.

When the brain map looks normal, the symptoms that brought you to neurofeedback should be greatly diminished."

Dr. Albright removes the leads from John's scalp. As he leaves the office, John says, "That wasn't as scary as I thought it would be. I actually enjoyed the session."

Chapter 3

Amazing Research Outcomes

The way to do research is
to attack the facts
at the point of the greatest astonishment.

–Celia Green

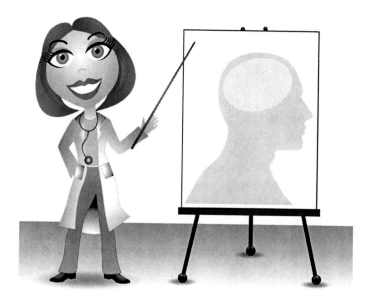

Neurofeedback has been quite impressive in one study after another. In fact, in studies conducted in its use for ADHD and ADD, it was rated as having a '*level 5 research outcome*'.

What does that mean? Perhaps the best way to describe the results of neurofeedback in the research that has been conducted thus far is to briefly explain the lowest level (level one) and the highest level (level five) of the five possible outcomes in a research study.

First, I will give the professional "text book" definition, followed by the "common household language" translation.

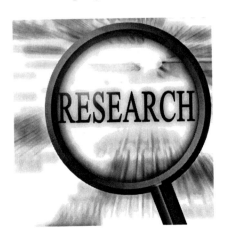

(Forgive me if I incorporate a little humor; we tend to remember things that are "odd" or "funny" more effectively.)

Level 1: Not empirically supported:

Level 1 means 'Mere Opinion' that the treatment is effective:

The effectiveness of the treatment is supported only by personal stories and/or case studies in non-peer reviewed venues.

Common Household Language Translation of a Level 1 rating of effectiveness:

Your Aunt Margaret tells you that rubbing maple syrup on warts will make them go away.

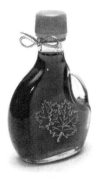

She's never tried it, and only knows about it because her Aunt Ruth told her about it when she was little.

Meanwhile, Uncle Charlie is claiming that baby powder will make warts go away.

What does this mean? It means that at this point, your Uncle Charlie's claim is on equal ground with that of your Aunt Margaret; there is no "proof" of either remedy working. *They are simply "Old Wives Tales" and little more than that, in terms of credibility and proven effectiveness.*

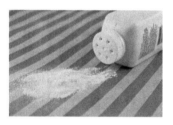

Level 5: Efficacious and Specific:
(Efficacious and Specific=Successful AND Specific)

The investigational treatment has been shown to be statistically superior to credible sham therapy (also known as placebo treatment), pill, or alternative bona fide treatment in at least two independent research settings.

Common Household Language Translation: *Your Aunt Margaret is a trained research scientist, who has conducted a study that showed maple syrup to be far more effective than a capsule with flour inside, a well known over the counter wart remover,*

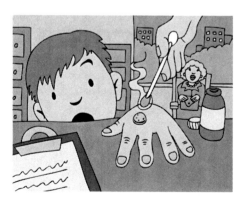

and a popular antiviral wart pill often prescribed by physicians. Another researcher, in a separate study, conducted by a different University, found the very same thing as your Aunt Margaret and her team of researchers.

(Neurofeedback Tip)

As well as some people do with certain prescription drugs, the results typically last only as long as the person is compliant, and takes their medication as prescribed. This is just one of the many areas where using neurofeedback differs from other methods of treatment.

Make no mistake about it, many lives have been changed - both the lives of people with ADHD and ADD and their family members - by prescription drugs like Ritalin, Straterra and Adderall, just to name a few.

As well as some people do with certain prescription drugs, the results typically last only as long as the person is compliant, and takes their medication as prescribed. This is just one of the many areas where using neurofeedback differs from other methods of treatment.

Studies have shown, time and again, that someone with ADHD or ADD who has been successfully treated with neurofeedback will continue to enjoy the benefits of those changes long after the treatment has ended. Some even argue, and research hints, that the changes may be permanent.

(Neurofeedback Tip)

Studies have shown, time and again, that someone with ADHD or ADD who has been successfully treated with neurofeedback will continue to enjoy the benefits of those changes long after the treatment has ended.

Furthermore, studies have also shown that neurofeedback is very effective for treating depression when used in conjunction with psychotherapy, and eliminated migraines in over 80% of those who were treated with this powerful new tool.

In the next chapter, we'll take a look at both the "pros" and "cons" of using neurofeedback.

Chapter 4

What Are the Pros and Cons?

Take a step back,
evaluate what is important,
and enjoy life.

–Teri Garr

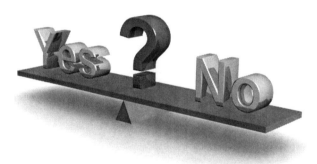

It has been said that there are "pros" and "cons" to everything; some argue that the cost of a clean-shaven face is a beard. It often comes down to a matter of perspective.

Here, I'll simply talk about the most common "pros" and "cons" and allow you to make the final determination regarding their significance for you and your particular situation.

(Neurofeedback Tip)

Pros:

Neurofeedback is extremely safe.

No significant side effects; in fact, side effects are very rare.

Results are long lasting.

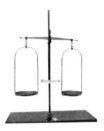

Pros:

Neurofeedback is **extremely safe:**

It's non-invasive. The electrodes are held to your scalp by a water-soluble gel that conducts the current coming from your brain into the EEG device.

No input goes into the brain; it simply reads the electrical energy coming from your brain. Understandably, neurofeedback is very safe.

No significant side effects; in fact, side effects are very rare:

People may sometimes feel a bit tired after a neurofeedback session. Body Language Expert and author of *The Productivity Epiphany*, Vincent Harris, reported that he was extremely tired after his 1st neurofeedback session, but that he was back to normal after taking a nap and getting a good night's sleep.

If you find that you are tired after a session, let your therapist know, and they can easily adjust the session to avoid much of the temporary fatigue.

Also, while very uncommon, some people may be sensitive to the conductive gel used with the electrodes. Again, simply let your therapist know.

Results are long lasting:

Because the brain is actually changing itself, learning to operate more effectively and efficiently, the results naturally tend to last through time.

If you put oil on a squeaky hinge, the squeak is silenced as long as the lubrication is present. If you want the hinge to stop squeaking permanently,

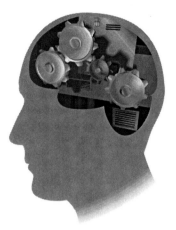

you need to identify, and then relieve the tension or pressure that is causing the excess friction. Once you do this, oil will no longer be needed; you have addressed the cause, rather than focusing on the effect.

⊂ Neurofeedback Tip ⊃

Putting a drop of oil on a hinge from time to time isn't much of an inconvenience; however, having to take medication everyday for the rest of your life may be less than desirable. Using neurofeedback is like adjusting the hinge and actually fixing the cause of the problem.

Putting a drop of oil on a hinge from time to time isn't much of an inconvenience; however, having to take medication everyday for the rest of your life may be less than desirable. Using neurofeedback is like adjusting the hinge and actually fixing the cause of the problem.

Cons:

Degree of change may be contextual:

Studies have indicated that when people use neurofeedback in the environment where the most significant challenges in their life has occurred, the neurofeedback results are even better than usual.

For example, if a teenager were struggling with being able to focus in his high school classes, where other teenagers are talking and creating distracting background noise, the results of his neurofeedback training would be even better if he could somehow do the training in this classroom environment.

Many companies are racing to create portable neurofeedback devices that will be easily able to address this issue.

Cost:

Neurofeedback sessions can run $100 or more per session. Assuming that someone can achieve lasting results with just 40 sessions, they are looking at an investment of $4,000.

With that being said, I have to tell you what one therapist I know asks his people to consider when he is talking to them about neurofeedback training.

After he has explained how neurofeedback works, he tells them,

"Before you decide to go ahead and begin the training, let me ask you to consider something. Pretend for a moment that we are 6 months into the future; you have completed 6 months of neurofeedback and have experienced significant and deeply profound results. In fact, you feel so much different than you had 6 months ago, that you sometimes feel like a miracle occurred."

He continues *"Now, if after you have experienced all of these wonderful changes, the ones you are enjoying so fully and completely now, thinking back to how much you had struggled 6 months ago, and I offered you $4,000 cash; I want to buy back all of the results you have achieved with neurofeedback, I give you the money and we just take away all of the positive changes you had experienced. Will you sell the results to me for $4,000?"*

He said he's NEVER had someone tell him *"Yes"* and that having looked at it from this perspective, $4,000 seems like a fairly trivial amount of money to invest in the happiness and increased quality of life that neurofeedback can bring them.

Most neurofeedback practitioner's offer payment plans for their clients. Some offer an interest free loan through www.CareCredit.com. In some instances, health insurance will reimburse a part of the cost of the therapy.

Now, in the next chapter, we'll take a look at how your neurofeedback begins.

Chapter 5

What in the World is a QEEG Brain Map?

"It is not down in any map; true places never are."

–Herman Melville

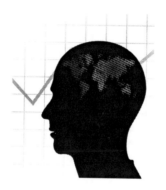

Anyone that has ever had the pleasure of staying at The Ritz-Carlton- a luxury hotel- will tell you that the experience is unforgettable. They are there to make you feel like a 'King" or "Queen", and that's exactly what they do.

Understandably, not everyone is working with a budget that will allow for such extravagance. And, even if they can afford to stay in such a posh environment, some people simply feel that all of the extra amenities are unnecessary, and are just looking for a clean room and a comfortable bed. The bottom line? They want a good night's sleep.

When it comes to neurofeedback training, a similar situation exists.

Some clinicians and practitioners require that you both begin and end your neurofeedback treatment with what is often referred to as "Brain Mapping" or a Quantitative EEG (QEEG).

If you have the financial means to do so, it certainly can't hurt anything to start with "Brain Mapping", but to assume that you can't be treated effectively without it, in most cases, would be a mistake.

Neurofeedback Tip

Some clinicians and practitioners require that you both begin and end your neurofeedback treatment with what is often referred to as "Brain Mapping" or a Quantitative EEG (QEEG).

With fees as much as $2,000 just for the "Brain Mapping", many people are happy to discover they can probably find a therapist who can get their baseline measurement for a whole lot less, using other methods.

Neurofeedback Tip

Two groups of people that would most likely benefit from having the QEEG or "Brain mapping" session; anyone with a seizure disorder or anyone with a traumatic brain injury should at least consider getting this initial assessment done.

There are, however, two groups of people that would most likely benefit from having the QEEG or "Brain mapping" session; anyone with a seizure disorder or anyone with a traumatic brain injury should at least consider getting this initial assessment done.

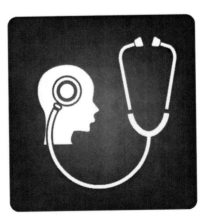

Just make a note to ask the therapist or clinician you are considering whether or not they feel your issue warrants the QEEG. Let them know that you have read that in some cases, it may not be necessary, and that if you can still be treated effectively without it, you may decide to pass.

I had my brain's EEG waves assessed for the first time during my first neurofeedback training class. The technician put the leads onto my scalp, and asked me to read a section out of a book. Then he asked me to count backwards from one hundred by sevens. He watched my EEG brainwave pattern on the computer screen with my eyes open and with my eyes closed.

I remember how tense I felt waiting for the technician to let me know the results of the assessment. He showed me how there were no epilepsy waves in the EEG readout, and how there were no 'sleep spindles' in the readout. He explained that sleep spindles show up when people are asleep, so it was good that none of them showed up in my assessment. He concluded that most of my EEG patterns looked good, but that my tendency to stay up late at night did cause signs of sleep deprivation in my EEG patterns.

Chapter 6

What Will My Neurofeedback Session Be Like?

Apprehension, uncertainty, waiting,
expectation, fear of surprise,
do a patient more harm than any strenuous exertion.

–Florence Nightingale

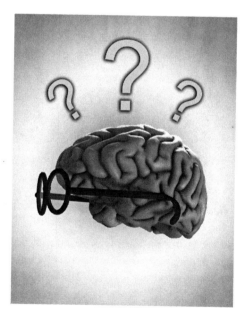

If you've ever found having a barber or beautician combing your hair or brushing your scalp relaxing, then you have some idea of what neurofeedback preparation is like.

Your scalp is rich with nerve endings, and most people find it very soothing and comforting when someone is gently touching their head and scalp.

Why would someone need to touch your head?

Very thin leads that conduct and transmit the electrical energy from your brain will be placed in various locations on your scalp.

A special gel is used to comfortably hold the leads in place.

After the leads are attached, your brain waves will be picked up and translated into something you can see on a computer screen, hear as some kind of sound, or feel through a vibration.

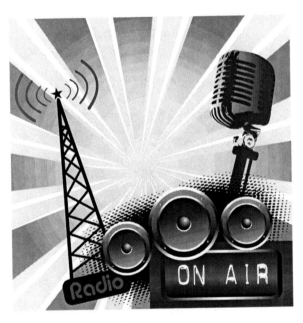

If you think about a radio, it's simply taking radio waves that are invisible, and then organizing those waves into sounds that can be transmitted and understood by those listening to a particular station.

Likewise, the leads will pick up previously invisible energy and then organize it into patterns that can be used to determine specific things about how your brain is functioning.

Once the leads have been attached, your therapist will have you alter what is happening to a visual on the screen of a monitor, like playing a game and moving a "Pac man" icon or flying a spaceship, for example.

In some cases, you may be asked to alter the tone or volume of some sound. You may even be doing both at the same time.

These movements, or changes in sound, are caused by your brain shifting into the desired brain waves; the very brain waves that will bring about profound changes in your thinking and how you feel.

Your brain interprets being able to change a visual or auditory signal, such as making the "spaceship" fly, for example, as a reward. Because your brain likes to be rewarded, it will seek to shift into the brain waves that bring about the rewards with greater frequency, and for longer and longer periods of time.

Naturally, these changes don't happen overnight; most people are delighted, however, to notice clear and obvious changes within the first 10 sessions, but to really etch the changes in and make them last for the long haul, several more sessions will probably be required.

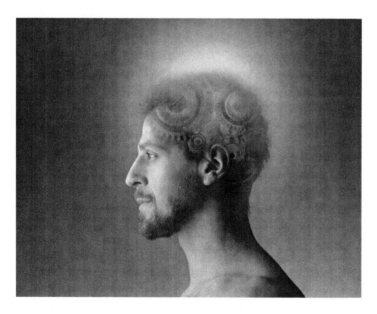

"How many sessions will it take?" is a frequent question from the many people who call my office each week. While I cannot give an exact number, I can say that some issues, like ADD, for example, might require 40 or more sessions. A Chronic pain issue may be completely resolved with only 20.

It really depends on the issue and the person being treated.

(Neurofeedback Tip)

If you feel nervous before your first neurofeedback session, you are probably in very good company. I remember the first time someone 'hooked me up' to a neurofeedback machine in one of my continuing education courses. I was thinking, "Oh no. What if they find out that my brain has problems that I don't even know about? This could be very embarrassing.

Luckily, all of my fears and concerns turned out to be unfounded.

If you feel nervous before your first neurofeedback session, you are in very good company. I remember the first time someone 'hooked me up' to a neurofeedback machine in one of my continuing education courses. I was thinking, "Oh no. What if they find out my brain has problems? This could be very embarrassing. What if I have a brain tumor from all that aspartame in the diet sodas I drank? What if they diagnose me?"

Luckily, all of my fears and concerns turned out to be unfounded. It was very interesting for me to observe my brain waves on a computer screen. Years have passed since my first peek at my brainwaves, yet I am still interested in putting the leads onto my scalp to take a look at how the ol' brainwaves are doing.

I remember the first time I asked my 11 year old son if he wanted to 'go on' my neurofeedback machine. He quickly said, "Yes". Then as I was about to attach the lead to his scalp I noticed that he became very nervous. "Oh no! Is it going to hurt, Mom?" "No", I replied. "Nothing is going into your scalp; it will just pick up on the activity coming out of your scalp."

Since I had 11 years of experience in watching my son's reactions to all kinds of new experiences, I was surprised to observe that his nervousness about the neurofeedback machine was in the top ten percent of his nervous reactions to new experiences.

(Neurofeedback Tip)

My 11 year old son began to fall in love with my neurofeedback machine after his first couple of minutes of neurofeedback training.

Now my son loves the neurofeedback machine. My machine has a setting where the client can operate a DVD with his brain waves. When the client's brain is responding in the desired way, the movie plays on the screen. If the client's brain is not responding in the desired way, the movie fades out. What 11 year old wouldn't like that kind of therapy? My son began to fall in love with my neurofeedback machine after his first couple of minutes of neurofeedback training.

Chapter 7

Neurofeedback for ADD and ADHD

I prefer to distinguish ADD as attention abundance disorder. Everything is just so interesting . . . remarkably at the same time."

–Frank Coppola, M.A.

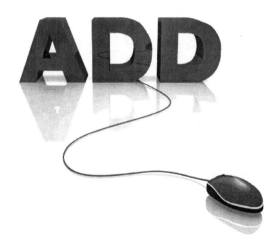

Attention Deficit Disorder and Attention Deficit Hyperactivity Disorder have quite a track record. Millions of young people and adults alike know the frustration and anguish that can go hand in hand with ADD or ADHD.

Happily, neurofeedback has a track record of its own; several studies have found that 8 out of 10 (80%) of those with ADD/ADHD who are treated with neurofeedback are able to leave the aggravating symptoms behind with just 30-40 sessions in most cases.

These studies have also found, that for many of these people, there is a measurable and significant gain of IQ.

In 1976 neurofeedback was investigated as a non-drug treatment for Attention Deficit Disorders at the University of Tennessee by Joel Lubar, Ph.D. Dr. Lubar's early work demonstrated IQ increases, grade level increases, and behavioral improvements for over 80% of the children in the studies.

(Neurofeedback Tip)

These studies have also found that for many of these people, there is a measurable and significant gain of IQ from neurofeedback.

Thousands of people quit smoking each year, just to avoid the negative consequences, like lung cancer, for example. Can you imagine how many more people would quit, if they not only could avoid the "bad" things, but could also enjoy a boost of 10 points on their IQ?

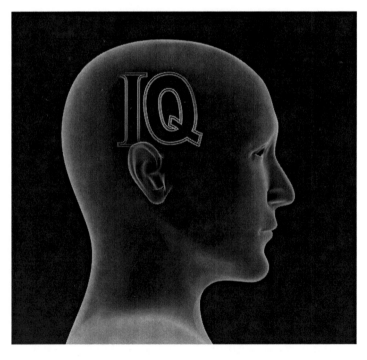

This is what *can* happen for the person who is treated with neurofeedback for ADD/ADHD. Not only will their ADD/ADHD likely become a distant memory, letting them move on with their life without the stress that often accompanies their previous condition, but they may actually be smarter as well.

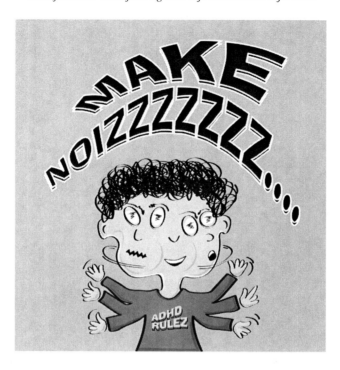

For the person who has suffered with ADD/ADHD for years, can you imagine how exciting it would be for them to wake up and experience each day like they had always suspected others around them did, but, because of the way their brain was functioning, those days had always been just beyond their reach?

Neurofeedback Tip

For the person who has suffered with ADD/ADHD for years, can you imagine how exciting it would be for them to wake up and experience each day like they had always suspected others around them did, but, because of the way their brain was functioning, those days had always been just beyond their reach?

I can tell you what it's like from my perspective. Each time I see a young life change, and watch their self-esteem blossom with the realization the way they had lived before will now be a thing of the past, I take time to step back and reflect on how fortunate I am, to have this wonderful and life changing technology (neurofeedback) at my disposal.

Chapter 8

Assessing ADD/ADHD with Checklists and a Continuous Performance Test

"I was trying to daydream, but my mind kept wandering."

–Steven Wright, comedian

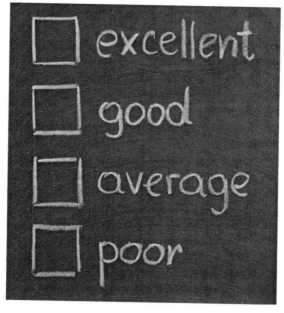

Until recently, providing adequate screening for ADD/ADHD was very difficult. For many years, the diagnosis of ADD/ADHD was made very subjectively. Clients were primarily asked a series of questions about their symptoms.

Clearly, this made the incidence of a misdiagnosis higher than it is today.

Fortunately, modern day technology offers a very rapid method for doing an initial assessment for the treatment of ADD and/or ADHD with neurofeedback. This modern technology is called 'The Continuous Performance Test'.

Three continuous performance tests now available are the T.O.V.A, the QIK, and the IVA. The three tests are very similar to each other. To explain this method of ADD/ADHD assessment, we'll take a look at one of these three continuous performance tests – the T.O.V.A.

The T.O.V.A. (Test of Variable Attention) was developed by Dr. Larry Greenberg. The T.O.V.A is a computerized assessment lasting about twenty minutes, (22.5 to be exact). It has proven to be an extremely effective and accurate tool for screening for ADD. (Dr. Greenberg was the Head of the Division of Child and Adolescent Psychiatry at the University of Minnesota)

People with ADD/ADHD often have a difficult time with anything that requires their sustained attention in situations they find dull or less than stimulating.

The T.O.V.A. is designed to present the person being assessed with a boring task. While they are taking the assessment, the computer is tracking their responses, and then comparing them to those of non-ADD/ADHD men, women, or children. It's no mistake that the assessment, or test, looks like, and is taken in such a manner that one might feel like they are playing a video game.

(Neurofeedback Tip)

Continuous Performance Tests, such as the T.O.V.A. is designed to present the person being assessed with a boring task. While they are taking the assessment, the computer is tracking their responses, and then comparing them to those of non-ADD/ADHD men, women, or children.

How reliable is the T.O.V.A.? In one recent study, the T.O.V.A. correctly identified 83% of the people who did *not* have ADHD, and 79%

of the children who *did*. The 8.3 and 7.9 out of ten people, respectively, are being identified far more accurately than the old subjective method could have correctly diagnosed.

(Neurofeedback Tip)

Just as the cell phone changed the face of communication all over the world, Continuous Performance Tests, such as the T.O.V.A has changed the way that many people are assessed for ADD/ADHD.

The T.O.V.A. is not limited to ADD/ADHD, specifically, though. It is also used to measure the attention of people with TBI's (Traumatic Brain Injuries).

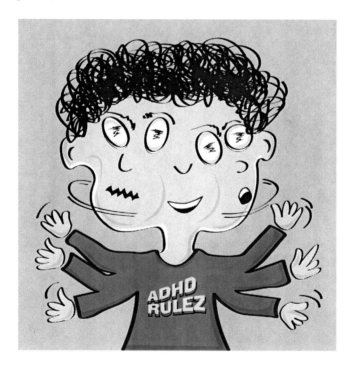

Just as the cell phone changed the face of communication all over the world, the Continuous Performance Test has changed the way that many people are assessed for ADD/ADHD.

Chapter 9

How Does Treating ADD/ADHD with Drugs Compare with Neurofeedback?

"ADD: Hunters in a farmer's world."

–Thom Hartmann,
from the book,
"ADD: A Different Perspective"

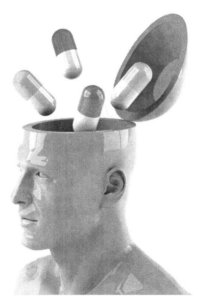

You have no doubt heard the quote that says if you give a man a fish, you feed him for a day. But if you teach him to fish, you feed him for a lifetime.

Neurofeedback is the equivalent of teaching a man to fish. Taking prescription medicine for ADD/ADHD is akin to giving a man a fish; in order to keep from starving, he'll ravenously consume your nutritional gift, too caught up in the satiety of the moment to realize that if you ever stop "feeding" him, that he will be as helpless as a fish out of water.

The current drugs prescribed for ADD/ADHD can seem to work miracles for those who have struggled with the issues that typically come with these disorders. However, with those "miracles" come a unique and disturbing collection of side effects.

In short, many of these drugs act as a legal form of speed, causing the brain (and other organs) to experience a stress response, so the person with a "muddled mind" can shift their brain waves back into the "attentive" and "awake" mode. It does work, but it can come at a steep price for many.

(Neurofeedback Tip)

The medications prescribed for ADD/ADHD are not intended to correct the underlying problem or cause of your symptoms.

More importantly, perhaps, is the fact that these medications can only relieve the symptoms for as long as you are taking them as prescribed. Stop taking them and you can almost guarantee that your symptoms will return.

Key Point: The medications prescribed for ADD/ADHD are not intended to correct the underlying problem or cause of your symptoms.

This is where neurofeedback shines. Neurofeedback is a treatment that focuses on correcting the problem responsible for the symptoms that many find so aggravating and limiting.

If you take a pile of cow manure, coat it with polyurethane, and paint it your favorite color, it will definitely *look* - and most likely *smell* - much better. However, the first time you poke it with your finger, you find, that, underneath, it's still cow manure, and it smells as bad as it ever did. Graphic? Perhaps, but in my opinion, it's no less distasteful than treating only the symptom, when in fact, a treatment for the cause is available.

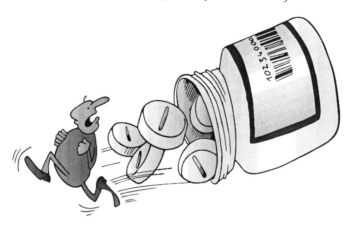

The real question is this:. Given the choice between having a significant improvement in your ADD/ADHD with side effects and a pill that you'll have to take every day for the rest of your life, or having the cause of the ADD/ADHD taken care of and a brain that self regulates, living free of the symptoms that you had experienced before, and not having to take any medication for the results you enjoy each day, which would you prefer?

(Neurofeedback Tip)

Men, women and children around the world are leaving ADD/ADHD behind and doing so without medications. How? Neurofeedback.

If you opted for the latter, you can consider yourself in good company. Men, women and children around the world are leaving ADD/ADHD behind and doing so without medications. How? Neurofeedback.

(Neurofeedback Tip)

Neurofeedback is a treatment that focuses on correcting the problem responsible for the symptoms that many find so aggravating and limiting with ADD/ADHD.

I should mention something here. There may be situations that warrant neurofeedback and medication. Just know that the two *can* work in conjunction if need be. And sometimes, this will be the case, at least initially.

As a mother I know that many parents would prefer a non-drug therapy for their child's condition. I am also a natural health advocate, who is always on the search for non-pharmaceutical interventions for the diagnoses and conditions that my loved ones are facing. Neurofeedback may be an avenue to explore alongside traditional stimulant medication to treat ADHD and ADD.

Chapter 10

Neurofeedback for Anxiety and Panic Disorder

"A panic attack is like drowning,
but there's no water to make you feel better about it."

–Anonymous

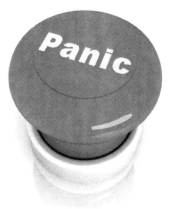

Every day, millions of people, in the United States alone, wake to yet another day filled with fearful thoughts and feelings, shrinking further and further away from the things they used to enjoy in life, and clinging to the security of their own home and environment.

Clinically, there are several differences between anxiety and panic disorder, even though the two are commonly used to describe the same thing. For our purposes, here, just know that panic disorder or "panic attacks" usually manifest very suddenly. Anxiety, on the other hand, generally builds up slower, over a few minutes or even hours.

Imagine what it would be like, if you were able to help produce, what many experts are calling a "cure" in 8 out of every 10 people who were suffering with panic disorder or anxiety, and do so within 30-40 neuro-feedback sessions. Would you feel obligated to spread the word about this magnificent tool? This exactly is what the available data is suggest-ing the "cure" rates are.

Neurofeedback Tip

Imagine what it would be like, if you were able to help produce, what many experts are calling a "cure" in 8 out of every 10 people who were suffering with panic disorder or anxiety, and do so within 30-40 neurofeedback sessions.

---

* When I use the word "cure" I am suggesting that the clients treated are free of 100% of the symptoms that had plagued them concerning panic disorder or anxiety. Realize that many different definitions of "cure" exist, depending on the organization or association commenting, and, some will even refute that a "cure" is possible. Call it what you like. Symptom free for months, even years, with no return of the previous symptoms is acceptable to me*

Please keep in mind, that millions of people have experienced sig-nificant relief in both panic disorder and anxiety with pharmaceutical intervention, including the use of medications like Valium and Ativan, for example.

However, once again, only the symptom is being treated. Unfortu-nately, most people experience a rapid return of their panic disorder or anxiety as soon as they stop taking their prescribed medication.

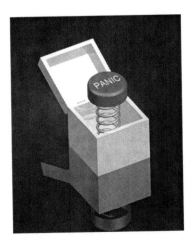

Furthermore, it is important to note, that drugs like Valium and Ativan (benzodiazepams) have been found to interfere with successful neurofeedback training. If you are currently taking one of these, and desire to begin neurofeedback, please let both your therapist and the prescribing physician know, and let them work together to switch you to another medication.

Neurofeedback Tip

When it comes to panic disorder and anxiety, I confidently move forward with my clients, knowing that they will soon be enjoying life to the fullest.

Over the years, I have felt the warmth and satisfaction that comes when a patient say's *"Dr. Albright, you are a genius! You're an amazing therapist."* Look, I'm human; comments like that feel wonderful, and, yes, I have studied my craft intensely for many years. In truth, however, I feel like I have been fortunate enough to incorporate some very powerful tools, and to learn from many gifted people. My primary tool, neurofeedback, has taken my practice to new heights.

I have made anxiety one of my specialties in the last five years. I have devoted as much time as possible to studying the different ways that psychologists can help people with anxiety problems. Of course, I studied Cognitive Behavioral Therapy, along with guided imagery, breathing techniques, and the newer 'energy psychology' methods, such as the Emotional Freedom Technique.

I even created an audio CD entitled, "13 Tools to Stop Your Anxiety Now, Without Medication", which you can purchase by contacting me at:

www.DrClarity.com

When it comes to panic disorder and anxiety, I confidently move forward with my clients, knowing that they will soon be enjoying life to the fullest. And, of course, singing words of praise about neurofeedback.

Chapter 11

Neurofeedback for Migraines

"If you have a lot of tension and you get a headache, do what it says on the aspirin bottle: "Take two aspirin" and "Keep away from children"

–Anonymous

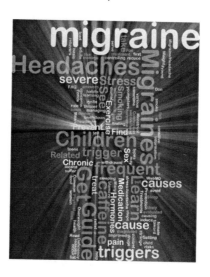

Very few people have never experienced the intrusion of a "simple" headache. For most people, rapid headache relief is little more than a couple of aspirin away. However, for those who suffer with frequent bouts of nauseating migraines, life can come to a grueling and agonizing standstill, and relief can, at times, seem light years away.

> ### Neurofeedback Tip
>
> 80%, or 8 out of 10 people who are treated with neurofeedback for migraines experience what many are calling a cure.

At the risk of sounding repetitious, (but I love repeating good news) I'll tell you, that, once again, 80%, or 8 out of 10 people who are treated with neurofeedback for migraines experience what many are calling a cure. We talked about "cures" a short time ago. Let's just say that the relief for those people appears to be permanent.

Research has shown that people who feel like much of what happens in their life is out of their hands, are more likely to suffer from headaches than those who feel like they exert a great deal of control in the outcome of each day.

Interestingly enough, neurofeedback is all about allowing your brain to take control by regulating itself. For the people who prefer the *"I'm the master of my fate"* belief, neurofeedback will seem like a natural fit. While it will work just as well for people who feel at the mercy of the world around them (neurofeedback works independent of one's beliefs) it may seem a little strange to engage in something designed to give them more control.

Neurofeedback Tip

Neurofeedback is all about allowing your brain to take control by regulating *itself.*

John Anderson is a neurofeedback practitioner at the Minnesota Neurotherapy Institute. He has been using neurofeedback for over 35 years. When I asked him about his work with clients with migraines, he replied,

"Most of my migraine clients get rid of migraines – either a great reduction in the frequency and intensity of the migraines or they get rid of them all together. I was recently working with one young woman who has frequent migraines. Before she came in to see me, she was having a migraine everyday and wasn't able to attend school. Now she's having maybe two migraines a week and is back to half-days at school."

Do medications work for migraines? In short, yes; for many people, pain medication has allowed them to once again participate in life. But remember, for a headache or migraine that packs a BIG wallop, you need a drug that does as well. By and large, the bigger the "wallop" the more significant the side effects.

My former spouse, Steve, is a victim of migraine headaches. He began to have them as early as age five. A few years into our marriage, we realized that the severe migraines were often triggered by consuming foods that contained the food additive MSG, or monosodium glutamate. I remember one day, Steve only touched an MSG containing food to his tongue, and he suffered a migraine headache that lasted three days! Needless to say, Steve has greatly reduced his consumption of MSG containing foods in the last ten years. Sadly, he still gets severe migraine headaches. I am looking forward to providing him with neurofeedback sessions in the year ahead.

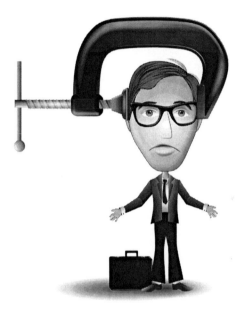

Do *you* know a friend or loved one that would enjoy waking up each day, knowing, and trusting, that they could breeze through yet another day in comfort? That they would no longer need to rely on prescription medications, or fearing that their plans would be ruined by a wicked migraine?

Why not share this book with them? It could quite possibly be their reality within a relatively short period of time.

Chapter 12

Neurofeedback for Depression

"Depression is the inability to construct a future"

–Rollo May

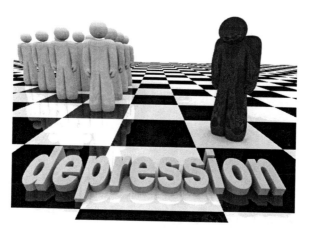

For the 25 years that I have been counseling in Orange County, CA, depression is the most frequent diagnosis that I see. My friends who are counselors tell me the same thing.

Perhaps the best way to start this chapter is by showing you some staggering statistics about depression.

- Up to 15% of those who are clinically depressed will die by suicide this year.
- The 8th leading cause of death in 1997 was suicide. The total number that year? 30,535
- The suicide rate among young people has increased significantly in the last few decades. Suicide was the 3rd leading cause of death in 15-24 year olds in 1997.

Clearly, depression is a very serious issue. Unfortunately, for many years, men, women and children around the world were hesitant to seek treatment, fearing that the stigma of psychiatric treatment would only add to their list of troubles. In 1972, Senator Thomas Eagleton's admission of having been treated for depression cost him the candidacy for Vice President.

Neurofeedback Tip

Unfortunately, for many years, men, women and children around the world were hesitant to seek treatment for depression, fearing that the stigma of psychiatric treatment would only add to their list of troubles.

Happily, many things have changed since 1972. Depression is no longer the "scarlet letter" of healthcare, and neurofeedback has proven to be incredibly effective for this condition.

Now, please keep in mind one very important thing; one of the most exciting things about neurofeedback for depression (other than the fact it works so well for many people) is that it is free of the burdensome side effects of some of the other treatments available.

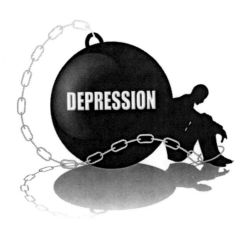

At the far end of the spectrum, we have electroconvulsive shock therapy (ECT). Anyone who has watched "One Flew Over the Cuckoo's Nest" will no doubt remember the graphic scene where Randall Patrick McMurphy (played by Jack Nicholson) received ECT. While not as popular as it once was, there are still approximately 1 million people a year who are treated with this method.

While I'm not making the claim that neurofeedback is a replacement for ECT, I would like to compare it with neurofeedback in a couple of key areas.

First, a 2004 follow up study of patients who had been treated with ECT found that as few as 30% of the patients had remission of their symptoms. More important, perhaps, was the finding that 64% of those patients would relapse in six months or less.

Next, patients who are receiving ECT have similar risks as patients going under general anesthesia. Furthermore, immediately following treatment patients may experience memory loss and moderate confusion.

Neurofeedback Tip

Enter neurofeedback. Those who opt for treatment using neurofeedback for depression are not only experiencing relief from their symptoms, but they are literally re-training their brain for long term relief and termination of those symptoms. And, of course, this is all done without side effects.

Enter neurofeedback. Those who opt for treatment using neurofeedback for depression are not only experiencing relief from their symptoms, but they are literally re-training their brain for long term relief and termination of those symptoms. And, of course, this is all done without side effects.

I've saved the best for last. Neurofeedback seems to work for depression, no matter how the person has become depressed. Meaning, whether their depression is the result of physical or emotional trauma; a genetic anomaly; or some other, perhaps unknown cause, many clients with depression respond very favorably to neurofeedback.

Chapter 13

Neurofeedback for Bipolar Disorder

"I still have highs and lows, just like any other person.
What I had with Bipolar Disorder
was a lack of control over the super highs,
which became destructive,
and a lack of control over the super lows,
which became
immediately destructive."

–Patty Duke, actress

Bipolarity is all about instability. The brain of someone with bipolar disorder is operating at extremes; at times it is seemingly stuck in a "funk", at others it is locked into "warp drive/hyper speed". These extremes can be seen on the EEG. When functioning in the "depressed" phase, delta and theta waves will spike. Conversely, when they are in the "excited" phase, we will see the prevalence of hi-beta brain waves.

> **Neurofeedback Tip**
>
> As I write, neurofeedback treatment for bipolar disorder falls short of being a "cure"; neurofeedback is used primarily to stabilize the patient. However, it should be noted that that there has been some success with completely cancelling the rapid cycling behavior that plagues so many with bipolar disorder.

As I write, neurofeedback treatment for bipolar disorder falls short of being a "cure"; neurofeedback is used primarily to stabilize the patient. However, it should be noted that that there has been some success with completely cancelling the rapid cycling behavior that plagues so many with bipolar disorder.

Understandably, this does not happen overnight, and may very well require more sessions than usual. Keep in mind though, the possible outcome is *full abatement* of the rapid cycling bipolar disorder.

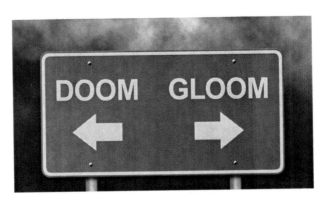

As a psychologist, I have been counseling individuals with bipolar disorder for over two decades. I have observed their frustration with the available treatments for this disorder. Most of the clients that I have worked with who have bipolar disorder must have medication changes every year to keep their brain and their life stable.

Imagine three large tubs of water. They are lined up in front of you; one in the middle, and one on either side of that one. The tub on the right contains water that is scalding hot. The one on the left is filled with near freezing water. In the middle, however, is a tub filled with soothingly warm and very comfortable water.

Now, imagine that you hop with both feet into the *scalding hot* water… OUCH!.. then you just as quickly jump back out…but land in the tub of *freezing* water…AHHHH!...now right back into the scalding water… OUCH!

The metaphor above will resonate with many who have suffered with bipolar disorder. Even though they suspect there might be a middle, far more comfortable, tub of water try as they might, they either find themselves in the very HOT or very COLD tubs.

With neurofeedback, you might say the patient is learning to cool the HOT water a few degrees, and warm the FREEZING water up a bit. Yet another way of looking at it would be the possibility of simply learning to spend most of their time standing in the middle tub.

No matter how you slice it, things are looking good when it comes to neurofeedback as a treatment for bipolar disorder.

Chapter 14

Neurofeedback for Epilepsy

"Epileptics know by signs when attacks are imminent and take precautions accordingly; we must do the same in regard to anger"

–Seneca

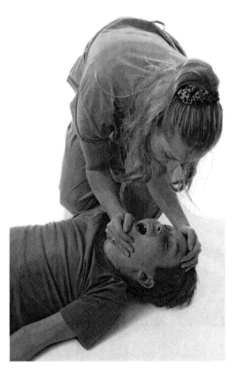

Not very long ago people were accused of being witches and burned at the stake, simply because of the misunderstood "firestorm" in their brain that unpredictably caused them to lose control; epilepsy was scary, for both those who suffered with it and those who witnessed a seizure first-hand.

Almost 30 years later, in 2001, Dr. Barry Sterman looked very carefully at all of the available research on the use of neurofeedback in the treatment of epilepsy. The results were very promising; of those treated for epilepsy - some of them experiencing severe and uncontrolled seizures prior to treatment - 82% improved significantly. There was a considerable reduction in seizure activity.

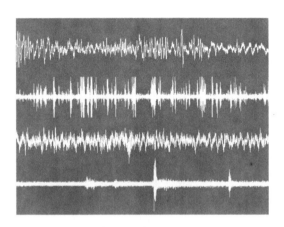

Now, knowing full well that the "naysayers" would jump on results like these, claiming everything from flawed studies to the placebo effect, one group of scientists utilized neurofeedback to do just the opposite. They actually wanted to cause seizures to be more intense, and to increase in frequency. Why? To show that neurofeedback could be used to train the brain in either direction. The results? They were just as successful going the other way-making symptoms worse-as they had been in using neurofeedback to reduce symptoms.

(Neurofeedback Tip)

Of those treated for epilepsy - some of them experiencing severe and uncontrolled seizures prior to treatment....82% improved significantly.

Were there still skeptics? Of course; we live in a society where some people still think the moon landing was a scam, and that Neil Armstrong was filmed on a soundstage, and not the surface of the moon. For some, the satisfaction comes from not believing. Fortunately, neurofeedback is one treatment that does not depend on the belief or expectation of the patient.

I remember one sunny Saturday morning when I was 13 years old. I heard strange sounds coming from my 16-year-old brother's room. I tentatively opened the door to his room and saw the horrible site of my brother having a grand mal seizure in his bed.

A few weeks later we were all playing a game of baseball in the school yard. At one point, when my older brother was playing second base, he lay down on the black top, had a grand mal seizure, and then stood up as if nothing had happened. The rest of us ran over to him in an alarmed state, while asking, "Are you OK? Are you OK?" He replied, "What? What do you mean?" It seems that he was completely unaware of what the rest of us had observed.

Neurofeedback Tip

I know first hand how troubling it is when a loved one has epilepsy.

I know first hand how troubling it is when a loved one has epilepsy. I wish that neurofeedback had been one of the therapies that my brother had available back in 1973 when this took place. Instead he had to take heavy medication that slowed down his bright conversational style.

Chapter 15

Neurofeedback for Autism and Aspergers

"I have a condition called Aspergers Syndrome, which is like a mild form of autism. It means I don't interact properly in certain social situations."

–Gary Numan, Songwriter/Musician "Cars"

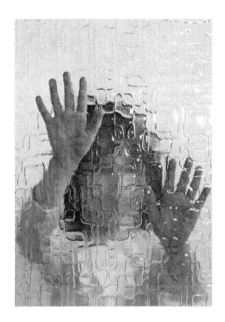

Autism is a disorder of neural development that generally manifests, in terms of visible signs and symptoms, before the age of three. We have yet to track down the exact cause of autism; however, most experts agree that there is a very strong genetic basis for this disorder.

Asperger's Syndrome, while being considered an autism spectrum disorder, does not impair social interaction or communication as significantly as autism. This is not to say, mind you, that Asperger's will not present obstacles; those obstacles will simply tend to be easier to function within society than those of autism. Some classify Aspergers as high functioning autism.

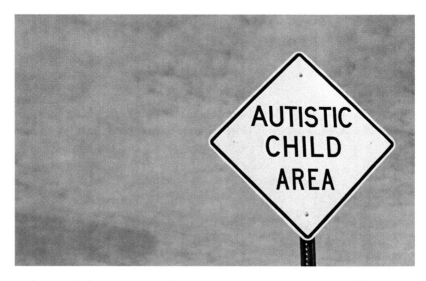

I learned about Asperger's syndrome late in my career. I have only had a good understanding of this disorder since the year 2000. It troubles me to think back on families that I worked with before then. Did any of them have a child or parent with Asperger's disorder? Did I miss something important?

Chances are good, that if this particular chapter has captured your attention, someone you know, is dealing with the challenges of Autism or Asperger's syndrome. If that's the case, you probably already know far more about these conditions than most people, and are not looking for a "What is autism?" manual; I suspect you are more interested in how neurofeedback could be used to change the life of a friend or loved one.

Let me tell you about a 14-year-old girl named Carly featured on 20/20 This little girl had been written off as being mentally incompetent. At a very young age she had been diagnosed with autism. For the first ten years of her life, she flopped and flailed and threw tantrums continuously. Her parents refused to give up and worked with Carly for 40-60 hours each week. Progress was minimal, but they persisted.

Then at the age of 11, Carly sat down at a computer, and lo and . hold, began typing one finger at a time. She revealed that there was a very intelligent young lady buried beneath the one she presented verbally and physically. She was not "stupid" or "retarded"; she was a very bright girl with feeling and emotions. She may have single handedly changed the way the world will view people with severe forms of autism. Carly is now writing a novel. (*I invite you to consider watching this clip on Youtube.com. A search of "Carly Autism 20/20" should bring it right up.*)

Neurofeedback Tip

Neurofeedback may very well be a tool that can bridge the gap between the human being on the inside, and the behavior displayed on the outside for those with autism.

Neurofeedback may very well be a tool that can bridge the gap between the human being on the inside, and the behavior displayed on the outside.

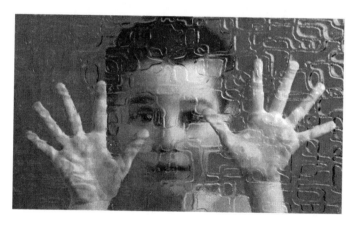

I'd like to share the results experienced by an 8-year-old boy diagnosed with autism; he had a very limited vocabulary, and did not like to be touched. After 98 sessions, the positive changes noted by his parents were:

- Medications were cut in half
- Memorized speech gave way to some original thoughts and ideas
- Speech patterns slowed down and became easier to understand
- He was initiating touch and asking for hugs

improvement in gross motor skills and balance
lity emotionally
nuch better with his brothers and sisters

The 98 sessions noted above would be typical of autism; the number of sessions needed may involve years, rather than months. And, I don't want to imply that the data exists at this point to support results like this for everyone using neurofeedback for Autism or Asperger's syndrome. I will point out, however, that no data exists to support the idea that it can't, either.

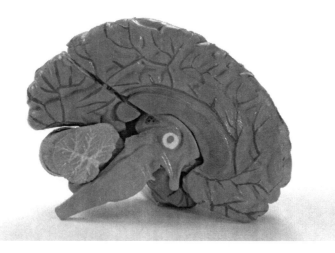

The results experienced by this young man and his family are "miraculous" when compared to other forms of treatment. A case like this certainly opens up a whole new realm of possibility and hope.

Case Study: Asperger's Syndrome

Neurofeedback Practitioner:
Dr. Gerald Gluck, Ph.D.
Coral Springs, FL
www.brainhealingcenter.com

I began treating a 10 year old boy who has Asperger's disorder about a year ago.

His parents are both physicians in Panama and they flew to Miami and stayed here for about seven weeks for the neurofeedback for their son.

I saw the child twice a day, four to five times a week for the neurofeedback sessions.

His mother had done a great deal of previous work with him, nutritional work, detoxification, and exercise. She was actually a pediatrician and had worked with him so that the child was prepared to work that hard.

When the child came to our clinic, his baseline was that he required an aide with him in a special classroom in Panama in order to get through the day, and he was in a cluster, an autistic cluster.

It's now been about a year since the neurofeedback sessions began, and when he returned to Panama:

• he was no longer in need of an aide
• he operated independently
• he began to make friends. He now has a social network of friends
• he now attends a regular class, and is actually
• participating in a role in the school play.
• for the first time in the history of their marriage, mom and dad were able to take a month and go to Europe and leave their son with a housekeeper. The parents felt that they didn't have to worry about their son because he was sufficiently independent."

Chapter 16

Neurofeedback for Treating Tourette's Syndrome

Tourette's: "There's a point in a friendship with someone with Tourette's ...where they ask, 'I've always wondered –
can you stop it? Can you, like, just stop?"

–Anonymous

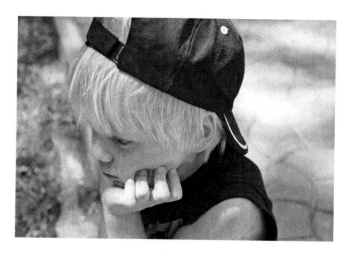

When many people hear "Tourette's" it often ushers forth thoughts of some seemingly out of control human being spewing an incessant stream of profanity. (The medical definition for this is *coprolalia*). In truth, the repetitious utterance of vulgar words is a symptom only found in a relatively small portion (10%) of those with the disorder.

As is the case with autism, the exact cause of Tourette's syndrome has yet to be discovered. There is, however, a significant genetic factor involved; a mother or father with Tourette's syndrome has a 50/50 chance of passing the gene on to a child.

One useful way of thinking about what's going on with the sudden jerks or "tics" that someone with Tourette's may suffer dozens, even hundreds of times per day, is to think about a lamp with a faulty switch. You touch the switch, and the light flickers on and off. Even the slightest touch will cause the light bulb to engage in an apparent dance of indecision, committing to nothing, but determined to do something - anything - until it finds itself doing something else. The point is, it's not the light bulb that's at fault, even though that's what is being noticed.

> **Neurofeedback Tip**
>
> In much the same way, we find the person with Tourette's (or the person sitting next to them) wanting to control the arm, the leg, the facial expressions or the mouth. But, in the same way that changing the light bulb would do nothing to fix a faulty light switch, tying the hands of someone with Tourette's, or placing duct tape over their mouth, would be just as illogical, and frustrating.

In much the same way, we find the person with Tourette's (or the person sitting next to them) wanting to control the arm, the leg, the facial expressions or the mouth. But, in the same way that changing the light bulb would do nothing to fix a faulty light switch, tying the hands of someone with Tourette's, or placing duct tape over their mouth, would be just as illogical, and frustrating.

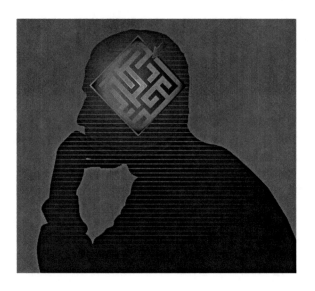

While we may not always be in a position to replace a faulty light switch immediately, occasionally just tightening the switch will get it to work. Sometimes the same is true for Tourette's and neurofeedback; clinicians may scratch their head in confusion at how quickly the symptoms have been reduced. Of course, there will also be times when clinicians are left wondering why things aren't happening faster.

(**Neurofeedback Tip**)

Try telling someone who was suffering from severe Tourette's symptoms, who is now able to seek employment or get involved in a relationship, only because they have made such marked improvements with neurofeedback, that there's not enough research to support it as a mainstream form of treatment.

Results are mixed, at this point, but try telling someone who was suffering from severe Tourette's symptoms, who is now able to seek employment or get involved in a relationship, only because they have made such marked improvements with neurofeedback, that there's not enough research to support it as a mainstream form of treatment. Given that the side effects are little to none, as long as it is financially feasible for someone to complete the needed sessions, why not use it?

Chapter 17

Neurofeedback for Dyslexia and Learning Disabilities

"I was dyslexic before anybody knew what dyslexia was. I was called 'slow'. It's an awful feeling to think of yourself as 'slow' - it's horrible."

–Robert Benton

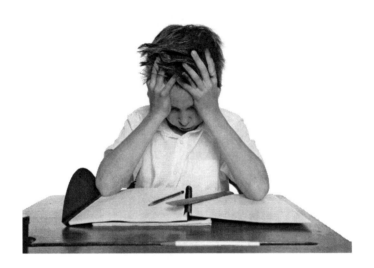

Imagine, if you will, a young child standing before their classmates, trembling inside, feeling stupid and deficient; they are struggling, not only with the fact that they don't know the answer to the question, or understand the concept being discussed, but with the inferior feelings that grow more intense each time the teacher puts their "ignorance" on public display.

I'd love to be able to tell you that this was an antiquated example; one that used to happen each day in classrooms from coast to coast. However, this is a pretty good description of what many bright young men and women face on a daily basis.

By now, I'm sure you have discovered my love for using metaphors to explain otherwise complex things. A metaphor is not meant to be an exact description; metaphors are used to show how one thing is "like" another, therefore, there will always be a gap between the metaphor used to describe, and the thing described. Now, having made that clear, I'm going to roll right into another metaphor, regarding learning disabilities and neurofeedback.

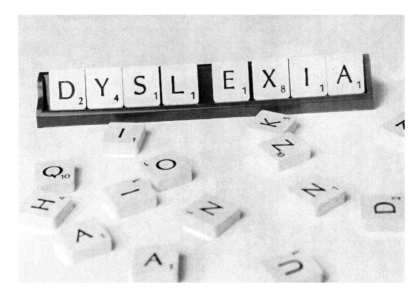

The brain of a child with learning disabilities is like a truck that is stuck in low gear, and a driver that has forgotten that higher gears even exist. It is exasperating to trudge from point A to point B in a grindingly slow forward crawl, while other vehicles are effortlessly passing you by. The driver never once considers that their truck could keep up with the others on the road if they restored its ability to shift into higher gears; instead, they beat themselves up for not being able to go as fast as the others, convinced they are already operating at their full potential.

> ### Neurofeedback Tip
>
> The brain of a child with learning disabilities is like a truck that is stuck in low gear, and a driver that has forgotten that higher gears even exist. It is exasperating to trudge from point A to point B in a grindingly slow forward crawl, while other vehicles are effortlessly passing you by.

Neurofeedback is a tool that say's *"LOOK! There are other gears you can use."* The first step is realizing that there are other gears (brain waves) available to you. Then, it's a simple matter of conditioning your brain to *choose* to enter those brain waves at the appropriate times.

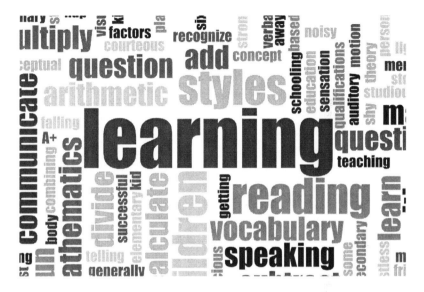

In 1985, a study was published about the use of neurofeedback for learning disorders. Researchers were startled by what they discovered. IQ scores in these children improved; there was an average increase of 19 points on the Wechsler - full scale IQ test.

Neurofeedback Tip

In 1985 a study was published after using neurofeedback for learning disorders. Researchers were startled by what they discovered. IQ scores in these children improved; there was an average increase of 19 points on the Wechsler - full scale IQ test.

In no way am I suggesting that all of those with learning disabilities will increase their IQ using neurofeedback. However, I'm not suggesting that they won't, either. My hunch is that even further jumps in IQ will eventually be seen using this wonderful tool for introducing people to their true potential.

Chapter 18

Neurofeedback for Treating Sensory Integration Disorder

No brain is stronger than its weakest think.

~Thomas L. Masson

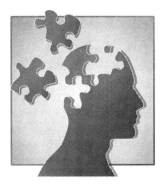

Sensory Integration Disorder (SID) was discovered by Jean Ayres, Ph.D. about 40 years ago.

As a psychologist, I am sad to say that when I was in graduate school, (1982 – 1987) that this disorder wasn't talked about much. At this time I am often involved with families who have a child with Sensory Integration Disorder.

Imagine, if you will, that for each of your 5 senses, there is a wire of a different color that leads the information from that particular sense to your brain. For example, for the information that comes in from your eyes, or your visual senses, you might imagine a red wire; and blue one for hearing (auditory), etc.

> **Neurofeedback Tip**
>
> When someone is dealing with SID, their brain is getting mixed signals.

Now, assuming that your brain was able to notice what color of "wire" the information was coming from, and knew that the red "wire" was information from your eyes, and blue was from your ears, it would be a fairly straightforward process for keeping things figured out. Someone with SID, however, doesn't experience it quite this way.

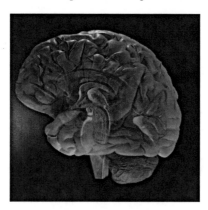

For someone with SID, their brain is getting the signals mixed . Sometimes the red "wire "might be visual information; other times, it might be the *blue* "wire" that is shuttling the visual data. Then, there may be times when the red "wire" is carrying *both* visual *and* auditory information. Can you see how this might be very confusing for the brain to interpret?

This sounds like a rather complex challenge, does it not? One could argue that it is, I suppose, but I've never been one for building a "case" for difficulty. Instead, I prefer to gather evidence for *possibility.*

In short, when neurofeedback is helpful for those with SID, it's as though neurofeedback is able to teach the brain to start recognizing the "wires" accurately and stop acting "color blind" when it comes to incoming sensory information. And, why shouldn't everyone's brain learn to clearly interpret sensory information?

Chapter 19

Neurofeedback Training for Treating Reactive Attachment Disorder

Having children makes one no more a parent than having a piano makes you a pianist.

-Michael Levine

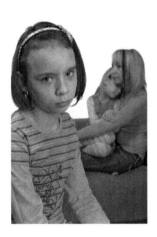

Sadly, not every child born into this world is held lovingly, wrapped comfortably in warm, soft blankets, and "oohed" and "ahhhhed" at by their mother, father, grandparents and other family members. And, many children, rather than looking forward to the ringing bell that signals "schools out!" at day's end, feel a knot in their stomach; they don't know what kind of chaos they are going to encounter, once again, when they get home from school.

Situations like these can lead to Reactive Attachment Disorder (RAD). When children fail to form the normal attachments to parents and/or primary caregivers, early in life, the "blueprint" they develop regarding relationships may lead to unnecessary conflict later in life.

Some of the most difficult cases that I have worked on in my 25 years of counseling have been with families who had a child with Reactive Attachment Disorder. Many of these situations involved a child who had been adopted. I would watch these children and wonder,

---

(Neurofeedback Tip)

When children fail to form the normal attachments to parents and/or primary caregivers, early in life, the "blueprint" they develop regarding relationships may lead to unnecessary conflict later in life.

- "Are you trying to reject your mother before she rejects you?
- Are you afraid that you are going to lose this mother, the way that you lost your birth mother?
- Are you trying to be 'in-control' of the loss this time around - by making your mother so miserable that you won't be taken by surprise if she rejects you?"

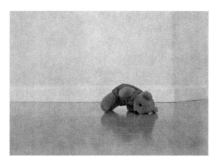

Studies have shown that in order for the part of a child's brain that is responsible for regulating emotions to develop normally, the necessary entrainment between the mother and infant's brain must occur during the child's first 18 months of life.

Think of "entrainment" as two people singing in harmony; when they are, it sounds beautiful; when they are not, it can sound like a cat with its tail caught in a mouse trap-not pretty. Brain waves in mother and child very often come into harmony with the brain waves of the other; they are in "sync" if you will. When this entrainment does not have the opportunity to occur, or, is for very brief and infrequent periods, proper brain development may be stunted.

The brain of someone with RAD is on high alert; it is easily triggered by many things that, in truth, do not represent any type of danger, but, because the brain interprets the event this way, the reaction is one that would be consistent with what we would expect if there really was some kind of threat.

(Neurofeedback Tip)

Brain waves in mother and child very often come into harmony with the brain waves of the other; they are in "synch" if you will. When this entrainment does not have the opportunity to occur, or, is for very brief and infrequent periods, proper brain development may be stunted.

Neurofeedback is used to reduce the arousal in the brain of someone diagnosed with RAD. When their brain learns to not become aroused (alarmed) as easily, there is often a significant reduction in aggressive and impulsive behavior. Clients will begin to willingly engage in, or even seek out, social opportunities.

(Neurofeedback Tip)

The brain of someone with RAD is on high alert; it is easily triggered by many things that, in truth, do not represent any type of danger, but, because the brain interprets the event this way, the reaction is one that would be consistent with what we would expect if there really was some kind of threat.

With a brain that now has the ability to more easily access the "calm zone" the person who was previously fearful in social settings, is now able to experience feelings other than fear - like comfort, pleasure and enjoyment - and start to enjoy the connections that often unfold when spending time with others.

Chapter 20

Neurofeedback for Parkinson's Disease

"I love the irony. I'm perceived as being really young and yet I have the clinical condition of an old man."

-Michael J. Fox

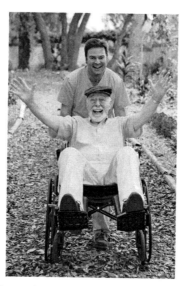

Parkinson's Disease has taken center stage in recent years after "Back to the Future" star Michael J. Fox and former Heavyweight boxing champion, Muhammad Ali went public with their diagnosis. Some 1.5 million American's are afflicted by the disease, with as many as 50,000 new cases each year.

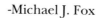

Neurofeedback Tip

According to experts, there is currently no known cure for Parkinson's Disease. Understandably, many doctors are very skeptical about the use of neurofeedback for Parkinson's.

When I was 13 years old my father began his 30 year battle with Parkinson's disease. His only brother is also afflicted with this disease. Since the disease is not thought to be hereditary, my family wonders if the heavy pesticide spraying in their hometown of Queens, NY, is involved in both brothers being afflicted by the disease.

If neurofeedback had been available to my family in the 80's, I think that it is likely that we would have invested in some sessions to try to ward off the crippling aspects of the disease.

According to experts, there is currently no known cure for Parkinson's Disease. Understandably, many doctors are very skeptical about the use of neurofeedback for Parkinson's. However, one aspect of treatment with neurofeedback they are not likely aware of, is that neurofeedback does not profess to correct anything in the area of the brain responsible for Parkinson's disease.

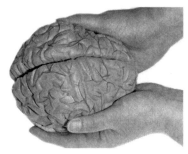

By the time the symptoms of Parkinson's Disease become obvious, some 75% of the neurons in an area known as the *substantia nigra* have been lost. This offers a great deal of insight; at the time of their diagnosis, most Parkinson's afflicted patients are still capable of moving most of the muscles of their body by willful intention.

Knowing that they are doing so, without, on average, 75% of these neurons, we can, by implication, determine that they are able to easily move at will *with just 25% of their substantia nigra remaining.*

Neurofeedback Tip

Since one major role of neurofeedback involves learning to better control and shift attention, and with each shift in awareness, subtle changes in what part of the brain is being used occur, neurofeedback almost certainly has a role in lengthening the period of time a Parkinson's patient can live an active life.

The human brain has a great deal of plasticity. This means that areas of the brain that aren't normally involved in certain functions will often contribute in a significant way, when the area that usually handles the task is damaged.

Since one major role of neurofeedback involves learning to better control and shift attention, and with each shift in awareness, subtle changes in what part of the brain is being used occur, neurofeedback almost certainly has a role in lengthening the period of time a Parkinson's patient can live an active life.

Chapter 21

Neurofeedback for Symptoms of Menopause, Pre-Menopausal Symptoms, and PMS

Women complain about premenstrual syndrome, but I think of it as the only time of the month that I can be myself.

-Roseanne Barr

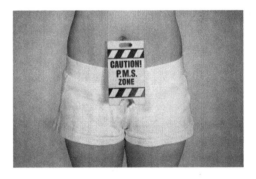

In my 25 years of counseling, I have been amazed at the percentage of my clients who have had serious P.M.S. each month. I have watched my clients seek out every known remedy in an attempt to avoid the stress of 'losing' one to two weeks per month to irritability, anxiety, depression, and cramps.

I have long been waiting for therapies that would come to the assistance of those suffering this predictable plight.

Pre-Menstrual Syndrome (PMS) has provided a near unlimited number of jokes for most everyone in comedy at one time or another. Both men and women tell the jokes, both men and women laugh at the jokes, and yet, as any woman can attest, when "that time of the month" has arrived, no one is laughing.

What research is showing, at this point, gives good reason for women around the world to cry...**tears of joy!** "Why?" you may ask, and I'll get to that in a minute, but first, we need to cover a couple of things regarding PMS.

(Neurofeedback Tip)

PMS has many things in common with depression.

PMS has many things in common with depression. Not too surprisingly, many women get some relief from PMS with the use of antidepressants. However, as is often the case, when using medication to manage symptoms, problems arise, once again, when the medication is discontinued. Medication, in this case, is doing very little to alter the structure or the origin of the problem.

PMS is all about disregulation; "out of whack" hormonal cycles that effectively introduce a further state of imbalance across and through many of the body's systems. Neurofeedback serves as a "regulatory committee" of sorts, allowing you to guide your cycles back into a state of balance.

(Neurofeedback Tip)

PMS is all about disregulation; "out of whack" hormonal cycles that effectively introduce a further state of imbalance across and through many of the body's systems. Neurofeedback serves as a "regulatory committee" of sorts, allowing you to guide your cycles back into a state of balance.

Sound too good to be true? If you've suffered from one nasty, agonizing cycle to another, month after month, year after year, it probably does.

Clinical studies, however, have found that neurofeedback can be nothing short of amazing for PMS. In fact, in one study, after 24 sessions, 9 out of 10 women no longer suffered from PMS in a way that interfered with their lives. Some women were fortunate enough to experience no symptoms whatsoever after completing the 24 sessions of neurofeedback.

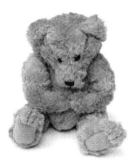

I should point out, that at this point no controlled research on neurofeedback and PMS has been published, but rest assured that it will be forthcoming. Keep one thing in mind; it's like the Wild West when it comes to neurofeedback. We are just beginning to understand the many different ways that this discovery can be used, and how many conditions it can successfully treat. It's an exciting time in history, to be sure.

Chapter 22

Neurofeedback for Treating Post Traumatic Stress Disorder – PTSD

"Fear is an emotion indispensible for survival"

-Hanna Arendt

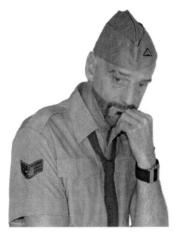

I believe that there are many people in North America who suffer the symptoms of Post Traumatic Stress Disorder and have no idea that they have the disorder. All that these individuals may know is that life seems hard for them, and that they never feel safe.

One of the saddest things about PTSD is that the effects of the disorder can negatively impact a person's life for decades.

Some of the best tools that I have to help my clients with PTSD are guided imagery, Cognitive Therapy, EMDR (Eye Movement Desensitization Reprocessing Therapy), biofeedback, and neurofeedback.

While fear has always received a lot of "bad press" and millions of people each day wish they could live a "fearless" existence, fear, and its corresponding thoughts and feelings, have probably been responsible for saving more lives than you can imagine.

We'd like to think that the real reason more people don't pull a gun and start shooting when someone cuts them off in traffic, is because of their own moral compass. However, more times than we'd like to admit, each day, the gun doesn't get pulled and fired, because someone *fears the consequences* of such a knee jerk reaction.

Neurofeedback Tip

In truth, fear is perhaps one of the most important emotions that we will ever have - at least in terms of our survival.

In truth, fear is perhaps one of the most important emotions that we will ever have - at least in terms of our survival - and to succeed in forever banishing such feelings would certainly bring about a much earlier demise than necessary.

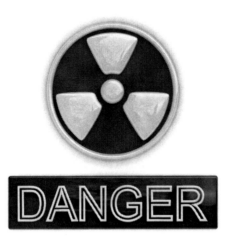

Fear, at the appropriate time and place, level, should be thought of as a guardian angel of sorts. When these fearful sensations are experienced in a time, place, and intensity that are not appropriate, however, not only has the "usefulness" of these feelings disappeared, but people's lives can get stuck in an aggravating and frustrating limbo of hell on earth.

Thousands of men and women proudly serving in the Armed Forces have returned, and continue to return, from the Middle East, suffering from Post Traumatic Stress Disorder or PTSD.

Neurofeedback offers a way to allow the patient to re-process the memory (or memories) that are responsible for their debilitating symptoms. Clinicians can, with the use of neurofeedback, assist a patient in experiencing a memory from a very detached place; almost like they are reading *about* the experience of someone else.

Think about some of the atrocities you have read about, or watched on T.V. regarding the Nazi Death Camps of World War II. As sad as it is to read *about* it, you can do so with a relative sense of comfort and security. Neurofeedback lets someone do the same thing with an experience *they have had*.

For someone with PTSD, each time they recall a certain event, it's like they are right back *in* the experience again. The goal with neurofeedback is to re-process the memory so they can remember it, almost as if they are watching this "other self", "over there", having *that* experience. In fact, maybe that's the best way to explain the shift that occurs; it goes from "*this* experience" to "*that* experience" in the mind and body of the person who has successfully re-processed the memory with the aid of neurofeedback. They can recall the information and relevant data *about* the experience or memory, without having to go through the emotions and sensations each time.

Neurofeedback Tip

For someone with PTSD, each time they recall a certain event, it's like they are right back *in* the experience again. The goal with neurofeedback is to re-process the memory so they can remember it, almost as if they are watching this "other self", "over there", having *that* experience.

Many people have already set themselves free from PTSD with neurofeedback. As the awareness of this wonderful tool reaches even further, we can offer this gift to our returning veterans, allowing them to move beyond the experiences they have endured, and to once again return to a healthy and happy lifestyle on the home front.

Chapter 23

Neurofeedback for Drug and Alcohol Addiction

"Just because you get the monkey off your back it doesn't mean the circus has left town"

-George Carlin

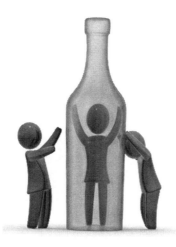

How successful is neurofeedback for alcoholism? One recent study found that 8 of the 10 participants did not drink during their 24 months of observation following neurofeedback. Interestingly, ALL of the participants in the non-neurofeedback group started drinking again during the same 24 month period.

Neurofeedback Tip

One recent study found that 8 of the 10 participants did not drink for the 24 months after the neurofeedback that they were observed. Interestingly, ALL of the participants in the non-neurofeedback group started drinking again during the same 24 month period.

In short, the neurofeedback helps correct the feelings that would normally arise during times of stress, by re-training the brainwaves to modulate at frequencies that are more consistent with a calm, non-stressed state of mind and body.

Just ask anyone why they started drinking again after quitting, and they'll say "The cravings!" When asked to describe "cravings" in terms of how it feels, it's not too surprising to find that the feelings are identical to feelings of stress.

Could it be as simple as no stress, no craving?

For those who have been so successful leaving alcohol behind because of neurofeedback, it would seem so. Ask them what they like most about drinking and they'll tell you "It relaxes me!" Again, in the absence of stress, we find none other than, you guessed it, relaxation.

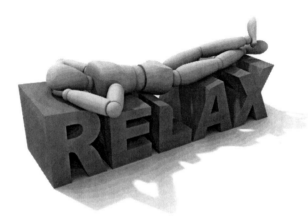

I know I didn't mention drugs one time; all I talked about was alcohol. Alcohol IS a drug, and people have struggled historically with the "quitting/relapsing" cycle with drugs like cocaine for pretty much the same reasons as with alcohol. You may hear that one drug is far more addictive than another, and at its core, that means that the feelings/ cravings are stronger.

(Neurofeedback Tip)

When the brain is trained to not experience stress in a context that it had stress before, where you once found a craving, you now find peace.

Remember the stress = craving formula? When the brain is trained to not experience stress in a context that it had stress before, where you once found a craving, you now find peace.

Too simple? Vernon Howard once argued that when it comes to what really works "the truer, the fewer" applies, and at least in this situation, it's very applicable.

Chapter 24

Neurofeedback for Treatment of Eating Disorders

"Often, a person will be anorexic for a while, then they discover bulimia and they think they are cured of the anorexia."

~ Terry Sandbek

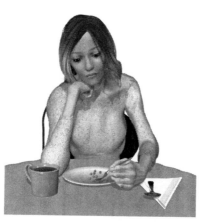

People with eating disorders like bulimia and anorexia, for example, are often dealing with such conditions as anxiety, sleep disorders, or depression at the same time. As you can imagine, focusing just on the bulimia, without addressing the anxiety or accompanying conditions as well, can be disastrous. It's the classic "Which came first? The chicken or the egg?" conundrum. Is the bulimia fueling the anxiety or is the anxiety feuling the bulimia? One thing is for sure; they are impacting one another, both of them are part of a system that coalesces to create the cluster of symptoms that plague them.

When used in conjunction with other methods of treatment for eating disorders, neurofeedback has the potential to radically increase the overall effectiveness of any treatment, and thus, a very favorable treatment outcome.

(Neurofeedback Tip)

Perhaps the most exciting aspect of neurofeedback is the fact that, when compared to other methods of treatment, for many conditions, the results tend to be far more resistant to change; something some researchers have even hinted at as being permanent.

As noted earlier, perhaps the most exciting aspect of neurofeedback is the fact that, when compared to other methods of treatment, for many conditions, the results tend to be far more resistant to change; something some researchers have even hinted at as being permanent.

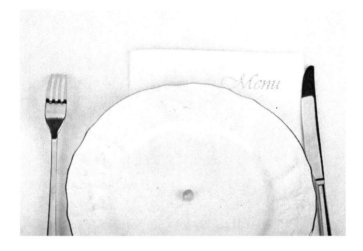

My first job as a mental health professional was working in an Eating Disorder Unit at a community hospital. One of my duties was to lead the group therapy sessions for the graduates of the program to support them in their after-care. During my three years working there we had 250 patients attend our program - patients with anorexia, bulimia, and morbid obesity. Twenty-five years later I am still working with eating disorder clients and their families.

It has been said that behind every behavior, there is a positive intention on behalf of the person engaging in the behavior. If we apply this to the person who forces themselves to vomit after binging, or the person who has become emaciated for lack of adequate caloric intake, and then ask *"What is the positive intention for behavior such as this?"* we might be surprised to find that we arrive, once again, at *feelings*.

(**Neurofeedback Tip**)

Getting thinner and eating less is to the anorexic man or woman, what nicotine is to the smoker; they are actions and behaviors that temporarily allow them to change their state of mind and body from feeling stressed to feelings of peace and relaxation.

Simply stated, the vomiting brings a sense of relief to the person who has just gorged on a large meal. Getting thinner and eating less, is to the anorexic man or woman, what nicotine is to the smoker; they are actions and behaviors that temporarily allow them to change their state of mind and body from feeling stressed to feeling peaceful and relaxed.

Anytime we can assist someone in moving from a stressful state to a calm or relaxed state without having to engage in potentially destructive behavior/s to do so, we significantly increase the probability for success. Fortunately, with neurofeedback, this is not only possible, but predictable as well.

Chapter 25

Neurofeedback for Fibromyalgia and Chronic Fatigue

"In 1995 testimony at a Congressional briefing (stated) that a Chronic Fatigue Syndrome patient feels effectively the same every day as an AIDS patient feels two months before death"

~Dr. Mark Loveless, Head of the AIDS and CFS Clinic at Oregon Health Sciences University

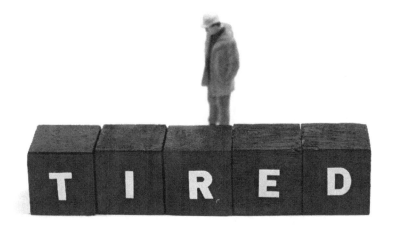

Fibromyalgia and Chronic Fatigue are notorious for destroying lives, but not in the way you think. Yes, the symptoms alone can push the strongest person to the brink, but for many, that's not what nudges them towards their breaking point. No, what many people find the most difficult to deal with is the doubt and skepticism - even by their healthcare providers - that anything is even wrong.

Can you can imagine waking up every day, your muscles painfully tight and knotted after yet another night of never having dipped into the stages of sleep where healing takes place.?

(Neurofeedback Tip)

Fibromyalgia and Chronic Fatigue are notorious for destroying lives, but not in the way you think. Yes, the symptoms alone can push the strongest person to the brink, but for many, that's not what nudges them towards their breaking point. No, what many people find most difficult part to deal with is the doubt and skepticism - even by their healthcare providers - that anything is *really* wrong.

As you force yourself to the edge of the bed, you pause standing, your muscles already burning, and the only thoughts on your mind (other than considering suicide) are getting to a scalding hot bath in an attempt to release some of the tension from your oxygen starved and aching muscles, and hoping that your hell like existence will either improve, or end. Lovely existence, is it not? This is the life of someone with Fibromyalgia. Chronic Fatigue is just as bad.

Now, imagine looking forward to feeling like this each day, too exhausted to even consider doing anything other than what is absolutely essential for your survival, and having your Doctor tell you "It's all in your head; your tests all came back normal." Sadly, this has been the experience of most Fibromyalgia and CFS patients.

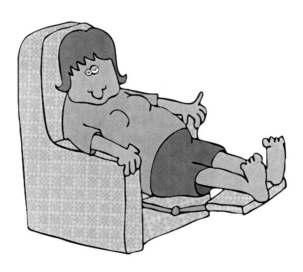

The muscular pain is often so severe with Fibromyalgia, that anything short of powerful drugs like Vicodin - even Morphine - does little more than add insult to injury. It's a double edged sword; to reduce the pain that keeps them from functioning normally and staying employed, the narcotics or pain relieving drugs, in the dose that's often required, renders the patient just as unfit for doing everyday tasks like driving or operating equipment at work.

Neurofeedback has been a godsend for many with Fibromyalgia. In one recent study, 7 out of 10 people who were treated with neurofeedback in conjunction with EMG and myofascial/craniosacral therapy experienced *total remission of their symptoms*. Let me say that again; *total remission, as in ALL GONE!*

Neurofeedback Tip

Neurofeedback has been a godsend for many with Fibromyalgia. In one recent study, 7 out of every10 people who were treated with neurofeedback in conjunction with EMG and myofascial/cranioscral therapy experienced *total remission of their symptoms*. Let me say that again; *total remission, as in ALL GONE!*

Results like this don't really surprise me. Many of those who are diagnosed with Fibromyalgia and/or Chronic Fatigue have a history of some kind of head injury. When the brain has been injured, one of the many challenges that will often surface is that of transitioning smoothly from one brain wave frequency to the next. A brain that is "stuck" in a frequency associated with fear and stress, for example, will eventually exhaust an otherwise healthy body to the point of being susceptible to a whole host of other problems. Both Fibromyalgia and Chronic Fatigue can spiral downward, seemingly out of control without the proper treatment and intervention. And, of anything I've seen for treating either one, neurofeedback appears to be more promising than any other.

Recently, one of my clients told me that when he was diagnosed some 10 years ago, his Doctor said of his CFS condition(?), "Well, you won't die from it, but you will die with it!" This kind of irresponsible conduct by health care providers does nothing but exacerbate an already trying situation. Fortunately, as it turns out, comments like that were wrong, and neurofeedback is a BIG part of the reason why.

Chapter 26

Neurofeedback for Stroke Victims

The brain is a monstrous, beautiful mess. Its billions of nerve cells -
called neurons - lie in a tangled web that displays cognitive powers far
exceeding any of the silicon machines we have built to mimic it.

- William F. Allman

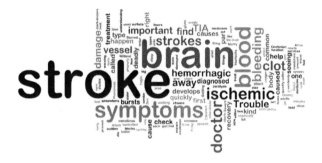

Stroke victims run the gamut; they range from those who have a temporary slur to their speech, to those who have been reduced to an existence trapped inside of a motionless body. And, of course, death is the
fate met by many, in the case of a massive stroke.

Stroke is the third leading cause of death in the United States. Most
people are aware of some of the more obvious complications that can occur after someone has suffered a stroke. However, there is one statistically
probable and debilitating condition that will often co-exist with the other
complications; depression often amplifies an already trying scenario.

Neurofeedback Tip

Stroke is the third leading cause of death in the United States. Most
people are aware of some of the more obvious complications that
can occur after someone has suffered a stroke. However, there is
one statistically probable and debilitating condition that will often
co-exist with the other complications; depression often amplifies an
already trying scenario.

Interestingly enough, studies show that the intensity of the depression is not associated with the degree of impairment brought on by the stroke. In fact, orthopedic patients - people who have had their mobility impaired to a more significant degree - will not experience depression at the same high rate as those who have suffered a stroke. This has led some researchers to conclude that the depression has more to do with the injury to the brain due to the stroke, rather than the restricted mobility.

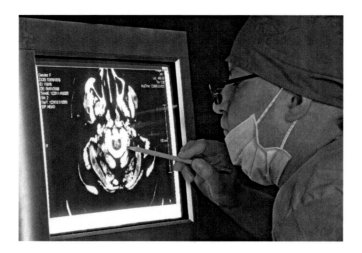

This is important for one very good reason. The risk of death is 3 fold for depressed stroke patients compared to non-depressed stroke patients, regardless of age, or type or intensity/location of stroke.

While it's an oversimplification, you might say that the person, who is immobile and depressed, simply loses their will to live, and this, of course, creates measurable and rapid physiological change that can drag the immune system down the tubes.

Neurofeedback is effective in stroke victims for improving balance, speech fluency, eliminating or reducing anxiety and depression, and improving attention. And, as I mentioned, successfully treating the depression in the stroke patient is of the utmost importance.

Neurofeedback Tip

Neurofeedback has is effective in stroke victims for improving balance, speech fluency, eliminating or reducing anxiety and depression, and improving attention. And, as I mentioned, successfully treating the depression in the stroke patient is of the utmost importance.

Clearly, physical rehabilitation and the like will be necessary components of recovering from a stroke. The discovery of the role that depression plays in a person's ability to recover from a stroke makes brain therapies such as neurofeedback just as crucial as physical rehabilitation in the treatment plan of the stroke victim.

Chapter 27

Neurofeedback for Cognitive Decline and Dementia

"I have seen deeply demented patients weep or shiver as they listen to music they have never heard before, and I think they can experience the entire range of feelings the rest of us can, and that dementia, at least at these times, is no bar to emotional depth. Once one has seen such responses, one knows that there is still a self to be called upon, even if music, and only music, can do the calling."

–Oliver Sacks

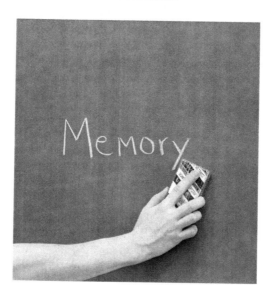

I remember, not that long ago, when an elderly persons mind started "slipping" and and they began getting things "mixed up" from time to time it was simply attributed to "Oh, she's just getting old!" In other words, it was thought of as some kind of inescapable consequence of living much past middle age.

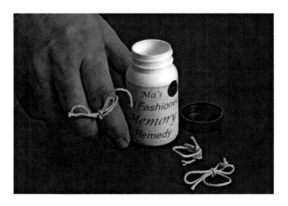

Our understanding of the human brain and nervous system, compared to even a decade ago, has allowed us to look beyond such pessimistic old age "sentences"; we now know that it is possible to alter the structure of the brain deep into the "Golden" years and much further, perhaps.

(Neurofeedback Tip)

Our understanding of the human brain and nervous system, compared to even a decade ago, has allowed us to look beyond such pessimistic old age "sentences"; we now know that it is possible to alter the structure of the brain deep into the "Golden" years and much further, perhaps.

In recent months a study looking at using neurofeedback to treat those suffering with the symptoms of dementia (such as memory loss) concluded that neurofeedback may very well slow memory loss, and, in some cases, may even improve memory.

(Neurofeedback Tip)

In recent months a study looking at using neurofeedback to treat those suffering with the symptoms of dementia (such as memory loss) concluded that neurofeedback may very well slow memory loss, and, in some cases, may even improve memory.

Granted, this does not sound as exciting as some of the previous chapters on the power and usefulness of neurofeedback. Keep in mind, though, that to even slow the memory loss and mental decline of a loved one - like a spouse - could be a very welcome possibility for those currently dealing with the deteriorating condition of a lifelong companion. Although research in this area is very limited at this time, future studies are sure to be close behind.

Chapter 28

Are Alzheimer's Patients Beyond the Reach of Neurofeedback?

I'm in awe of people out there who deal with Alzheimer's, because they have to deal with death 10 times over, year after year.

-Marcia Wallace

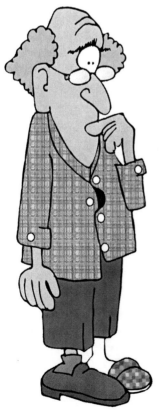

Society has a tendency to assume the worst possible outcomes about things that are not clearly understood. The lack of understanding translates into a lack of perceived control, and, when we feel like we have little to no control, we give up, rather than fight. This is where many families are with Alzheimer's; they have watched a family member drift mentally, farther and farther away, until suddenly, it seems that all that is left is a fleshy shell that bears resemblance of a once vibrant human being.

Professor John Gruzelier, from Imperial College London at Charing Cross hospital has commented *"Neurofeedback has been proven to be effective in altering brain activity, but the extent to which such alterations can influence behavior are still unknown."* Notice, he did not place a cap on what is possible, he is simply saying, in so many words *"this much we know, and we need to see what else there is to know"*

How does neurofeedback help with Alzheimer's disease? The method for using neurofeedback is the same as it is for anything else, but the specifics of what, exactly, is changing when someone improves, is hard to pin down. The reason is quite simple; Alzheimer's disease is not fully understood in terms of how it manifests and what causes it to progress. There is still a great deal more to discover about this malady before we can talk definitively about what happens to whom, and when.

Neurofeedback Tip

Society has a tendency to assume the worst possible outcomes about things that are not clearly understood. The lack of understanding translates into a lack of perceived control, and, when we feel like we have little to no control, we give up, rather than fight. This is where many families are with Alzheimer's.

What we can say at this point, is that many case studies exist that demonstrate neurofeedback's ability to initiate positive changes in people who have been diagnosed with this condition. Some of them are very remarkable changes; others are far less impressive, but positive changes nonetheless. As we begin to discover more about what is happening within the brain of those who suffer with Alzheimer's, we will be able to more accurately determinehow to best use neurofeedback to intervene.

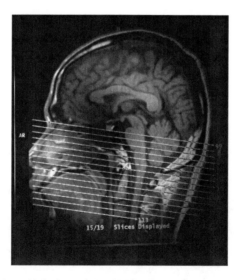

I began studying Alzheimer's in 1987 when I was in a Geriatric Internship funded by the National Institute of Mental Health. I was able to get training from some of the leading psychologists at UCLA's Neuropsychiatric Institute. I am hoping that as the decades go by there will be more and more tools to help individuals and families who are afflicted with Alzheimer's disease.

(**Neurofeedback Tip**)

As we begin to discover more about what is happening within the brain of those who suffer with Alzheimer's, we will be able to more accurately determine how to best use neurofeedback to intervene.

Chapter 29

Neurofeedback for Traumatic Brain Injuries And Post Concussive Syndrome

"No head injury is too severe to despair of,
nor too trivial to ignore."

- Hippocrates

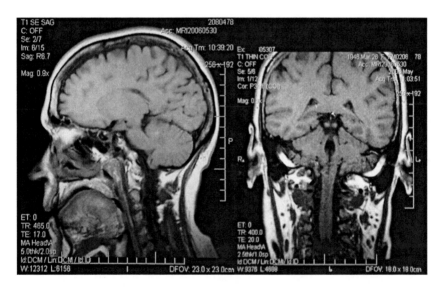

When most people think about a traumatic brain injury (TBI) it conjures images of someone lying near some scene of horrific carnage-blood and debris running and scattered about - a ragged body being carted off by paramedics. While tragic scenarios like this certainly occur each day, hundreds of thousands of men, women and children suffer a

TBI that may appear to be little more than an innocent "bump on the noggin!"

Neurofeedback Tip

Hundreds of thousands of men, women and children suffer a TBI each day that may appear to be little more than an innocent "bump on the noggin!"

Your skull is an incredibly effective protective casing for a gelatinous glob of goo that orchestrates everything that goes on in your life-your brain. The "hard shell around soft stuff" structure is adequate for many situations, however, one thing this design did not account for millions of years ago, was the rapid deceleration of a body that has been moving at 70 mph, that, in a few tenths of a second, comes to a complete STOP!

In fact, it didn't even account for this at 35 mph (a speed where a great many automobile accidents and TBI's occur). When sudden stops like this happen, the brain SLAMS into the bony structure that evolved to protect it. As you might imagine, the brain was not designed with such an event in mind.

Body language expert and author of *The Productivity Epiphany*, Vincent Harris was nearly beaten to death late one night in San Diego, California in the mid 90's. Unconscious for several hours, it was obvious to physicians - and later to Vince - that he had sustained a serious head injury.

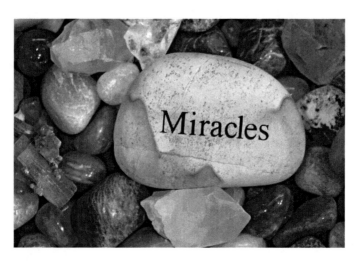

What Vince had never considered or been informed of, however, wi that when he was knocked unconscious for a few seconds playing high school football, and had his "bell rung" repeatedly in the 40 plus street fights he was in as an out of control and angry teenager, he had suffered a variety of brain injuries in these instances as well. Brain injuries can even occur from some seemingly insignificant events.

By clinical definition brain injuries are classified by placing them in one of three grades of severity.

Grade I: A concussion resulting in a short period of confusion (up to 15 minutes)

Grade II: Concussion that results in amnesia directly related to the confusion without loss of consciousness (lasting more than 15 minutes)

Grade III: Loss of consciousness with post-traumatic amnesia that lasts from 1- 24 hours.

As you can see, the first two classifications do *not* require the person to have lost consciousness. Almost every child that has boxed has, at some point, suffered from a Grade I brain injury. Suffice it to say that most people have no idea how easily TBI's can, and do, occur.

Fortunately, those who have suffered a TBI usually respond powerfully and quickly to neurofeedback. If prior to the TBI, the patient had been high functioning, and not dealing with some of the other issues presented thus far in previous chapters, the available data suggest that patients may return to their pre-injury level of function in 10 neurofeedback sessions or less. If you have suffered a TBI and are experiencing symptoms that are related to your injury, you may want to call me for an appointment if you live in the area, or seek another highly skilled neurofeedback clinician, because significant progress is likely.

(Neurofeedback Tip)

Case studies show that, among other things, patients are delightfully surprised to see a return of their short term memory, ability to organize, prioritize and sequence, and overall, get a sense of things being normal again.

s show that, among other things, patients are delightfully see a return of their short term memory, ability to organize, d sequence, and overall, get a sense of things being normal again, a. the appropriate number of neurofeedback sessions.

Case Study: Post Concussive Syndrome

Client - Jenn, Age 37

"I was in a car accident three years ago and since then, my life has been completely different.

I don't think there's one part of my life that is the same anymore.

I was diagnosed with persistent post-concussive syndrome after two years and three months, when the doctors realized that I was not going to take antidepressants and shut up about what was going on with me.

- I wanted to know what my symptoms were about.
- I wanted to know why I was throwing up.
- I wanted to know why I hadn't slept in three years, or two years at the time.
- I wanted to know why I had a headache.
- I wanted to know why I was severely depressed.
- I wanted to know why I didn't remember months at a time.
- I wanted to know what everything was about, and every response I received from doctors was that I was so high-functioning, nobody could help me or that nothing was wrong.

We've since found out that my IQ dropped from 131 to 121. And even though my test results show that I was in the 98th percentile on some tests, on other tests, I tested at 25% IQ, while at the same time, the doctors were saying "she has no cognitive problems. It's depression. She's a female, she's depressed".

I'd say, "I can't multi-task…everything coming at me all at once - I can't handle that, when I used to handle a multitude of things".

I was an attorney, licensed in two states. I used to prosecute drunk driving cases, sometimes 60 cases a day in court, without batting an eye.

And now I was unable to speak on the phone and write down an appointment at the same time. And doctors were telling me I needed to just take antidepressants because I had 'no cognitive issue'.

I set up an appointment with Dr. Victoria Ibric, M.D. in Pasadena, went in, and did some tests. I'd see all these pictures with pretty colors on the QEEG (Quantitative EEG) and I'd say, "Well, explain to me. Why can't I set up an appointment and talk on the phone at the same time?" She said, "See this picture? See how it's all red? That's why you can't, because that part of your brain is not communicating. The parts of your brain there that give you the ability to make an appointment and talk on the phone at the same time...see how those parts are red? They're not working.

Then Dr. Ibric started me on one round of neurofeedback, and I slept for the first time for five hours.

The thing with neurofeedback, for me, is parts of my brain were either communicating way too fast or way too slow, and that's called coherence. Coherence is the connection between two parts of the brain.

I also bought some equipment to do neurofeedback at home. But unfortunately it was too complicated for me to really be able to figure out how to do it.

I did another round of neurofeedback, and the results have been astounding. I read a newspaper article for the first time in years, and I understood the sentences, what the words were together, and could understand the sentences and the paragraphs.

I've had 74 sessions of neurofeedback. My brain was big-time 'off'. I mean, I was testing in the 35 percentile on parts of my brain, while other parts of my brain were functioning at 98%. My brain coherence was massively off.

The headaches are a lot more manageable. So many of my symptoms are subsiding. I'm happy.

The results of the neurofeedback are sticking. So it's not like these are getting better and then subsiding; a lot of this is actually sticking.

People need to know about this because there's no need for people to live in the hell that post concussive syndrome is. Because you look fine on the outside, non-visible injuries have a dynamic that is so difficult for people to be compassionate about and to understand."

Chapter 30

Neurofeedback for Managing Chronic Pain

""Pain is such an uncomfortable feeling that even a tiny amount of it is enough to ruin every enjoyment."

~ Will Rogers

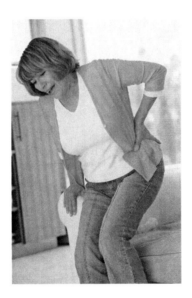

I'm going to make a bold statement in just a moment, a statement, that, if you are now suffering with Chronic pain may rub you the wrong way - initially. However, you might do well to realize that this statement is not only backed by new discoveries in neuroscience, but it also holds the key to bringing your nightmare with chronic pain to a very possible end. Here we go:

All Pain Occurs in the Brain!

Oh, I know, people have the *experience* of pain from just about every known location on the human body; this pain, and the perception of where it is coming from is very real to the person feeling it, but, that does not change the fact that *all pain occurs in the brain.*

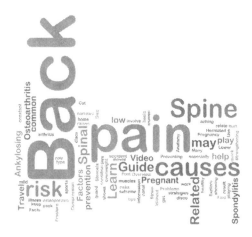

Excitingly, researchers have reported that many of their findings point to many instances of chronic pain as being like a "ghost"; an ethereal image of something that once was, but is no more. The problem with a "ghost" at least in the Hollywood depiction is that the "ghost's" do not know they are dead. The unfortunate mortals that happen to encounter a "ghost" are scared nonetheless.

Neurofeedback Tip

Oh, I know, people have the *experience* of pain from just about every known location on the human body; this pain and the perception of where it is coming from is very real to the person feeling it, and, that does not change the fact that *all pain occurs in the brain.*

Once the "ghost" becomes aware of the fact that it is trapped between its former plane of existence, and the afterlife, and clearly understands that it no longer has a role on earth, it dissipates into nothingness.

Chronic pain is often the same. Perhaps there was an injury, to a shoulder, for example, at some time in the past. It was a legitimate injury;

tissue was damaged, and the appropriate healing response, in terms of inflammation (which comes with varying degrees of pain) ensued.

Over time, however, and long after the shoulder injury had healed, the memory of those pain signals are still trapped in a ghost like existence within the nervous system of the person who is now enduring a pain that has outlived its usefulness.

Once a physician or healthcare provider has confirmed that there is no longer an injury, or that a previous injury has healed completely, and yet, you are still experiencing pain in that area, you are probably a very good candidate for being treated with neurofeedback, and for experiencing partial - or even complete - relief after being treated with the needed sessions.

Narcotics, with all of the temporary (and much needed) relief they can deliver, do nothing to release the "ghost" pain signals from the brain and nervous system. One reason that hypnosis has proved so useful for various types of pain in the past is that, once again, the pain occurs in the brain. Therefore, when the "maps" that are being used by the brain concerning pain are altered using hypnosis, patients often experience a 100% recovery from that pain, even with pain that had not responded well to narcotics and other forms of treatment.

(Neurofeedback Tip)

Therefore, when the "maps" that are being used by the brain concerning pain are altered using hypnosis, patients often experience a 100% recovery from that pain, even with pain that had not responded well to narcotics and other forms of treatment.

You may want to think of neurofeedback as a step up from hypnosis, or, maybe you won't. Maybe you'd just like to discover whether it will be as effective for you or a loved one, as it has been for so many others. No matter how you choose to think about chronic pain and neurofeedback, the fact is that lives are being changed by it every day, and people are once again returning to a normal life with this wonderful tool.

Chapter 31

Neurofeedback for Improving your Golf Game

"Golf is a game that is played on a five-inch course - the distance between your ears"

-Bobby Jones

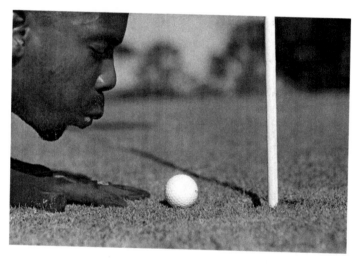

Golfers are notorious for being fanatical about doing whatever may be required to sharpen their game. While a mental aspect is present in virtually every known sport, one would be hard pressed to find an athletic activity where the "head game" plays a bigger part than it does with golf.

At its core, all neurofeedback training is *relaxation* training.

Regardless of the brain region or frequencies that are being trained, there is a component of relaxation involved. By allowing the brain to relax, it is feasible to train precise changes in brain state in very exacting locations, and in very specific ways.

> **(Neurofeedback Tip)**
>
> When a golfer learns to access certain states of mind, the ability to get into the "zone" at will naturally takes his or her golf game to a whole new level.

Neurofeedback never pushes for anything to occur; neurofeedback simply tells the brain when the desired state is happening. When a golfer learns to access certain states of mind, the ability to get into the "zone" at will naturally takes his or her golf game to a whole new level.

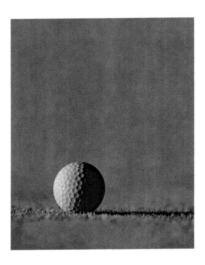

Almost every long-time golfer has experienced, the "Yips" at least once in their life. The "Yips" is a golf phenomenon that involves "freezing" while putting. Dr. Aynsley Smith, Director of Sports Psychology and Sports Medicine at Mayo Clinic, is convinced that the "Yips" likely have physical *and* psychological underpinnings.

The problem with doing things like taking a deep breath, or trying to relax just before, or during a putt, is that this requires the golfer to involve their conscious mind, potentially distracting them from the ability to focus. Neurofeedback, on the other hand, allows a golfer to make the ability to shift into the appropriate brain waves and state of mind an automatic process.

One advantage of using neurofeedback to improve your golf game is that you will most assuredly experience pleasant and positive shifts in other areas and contexts as well. Will it be your golf game AND your sleep that improve, or will it be your golf game AND your energy levels?

Neurofeedback Tip

The problem with doing things like taking a deep breath, or trying to relax just before, or during a putt, is that this requires the golfer to involve their conscious mind, potentially distracting them from the ability to focus. Neurofeedback, on the other hand, allows a golfer to make the ability to shift into the appropriate brain waves and state of mind an automatic process.

While I can't know for sure, I can certainly predict, that whatever other areas they are, you'll enjoy these changes just as much as you enjoy taking a few strokes off your golf game. Well, maybe not quite *that* much, but after all, what can be better than an improved golf game for a golfer?

Chapter 32

Neurofeedback for Peak Performance

"The successful warrior is the average man, with laser-like focus."

~Bruce Lee

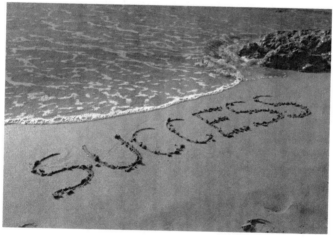

Peak performance is all about being at your best whenever you choose to be at your best. You've had those moments when everything was clicking; when everything you looked at was crisp and clean; when the clarity of what you were hearing was like you were in a recording studio, and the sensations that normally escaped your awareness were buzzing with a comforting strength, making their way into your conscious experience.

As a Peak Performance Coach, my job is to assist my clients in being able to dial into these states anytime they choose, and while I'd like to be able to take *all* the credit each time this happens, I have to admit, neurofeedback - this wonderful tool - is a big part of the results my clients experience.

One of my favorite parts of my work week is being on the phone, coaching my peak performance clients. I was able to attend two coaching schools after I finished my degree in Clinical Psychology. I can use Skype, a free video telephone internet service, to coach clients all over the world.

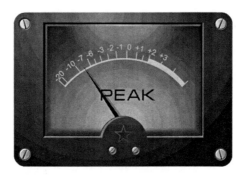

Common areas where people are seeking to be able to quickly and easily tap into a peak performance state of mind and body are:

- **Business**
- **Sales**
- **Therapists**
- **Athletes**
- **Managers**
- **Parents**
- **Students**
- **Artists**
- **Writers**
- **Surgeons**
- **And much, much more**

(**Neurofeedback Tip**)

Being able to operate at your best, reliably and consistently is not reserved for the elite.

Being able to operate at your best, reliably and consistently is not reserved for the elite. What if you could step into the feeling that you may have only experienced once in your life, of being a completely calm, loving, and in-control parent, even when chaos was happening all around you? With neurofeedback, it's possible.

Can you imagine being as razor sharp, with every cli
sion, as you have experienced only a handful of blissfu
past? Once again, with neurofeedback, this outcome is feasi.
more importantly, very useful *for both you and your clients.*

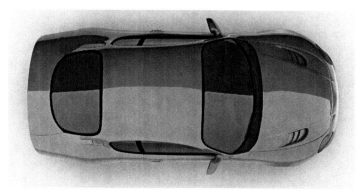

Are you a top salesperson in your company? If so, why not shatter your previous records and help even more people, putting a big chunk of additional cash in the bank this year while you're at it?

(Neurofeedback Tip)

The key with using neurofeedback for peak performance is that, most of the time, there was nothing *wrong* to begin with; you are not using neurofeedback to correct a "problem", you are only taking something that was already working well, and making it work even better!

The key to using neurofeedback for peak performance is that, most of the time, there is nothing *wrong* to begin with; you are not using neurofeedback to correct a "problem", you are only taking something that was already working well, and making it work even better!

Case Study: Edie's story – Neurofeedback and Meditation

At age 59, Edie had extensive experience with meditating, and felt that she had successfully "peeled the layers of the onion" in counseling. Still, Edie had a sense that she could accomplish so much more.

"By the time you get to be about sixty," she says, "what you're left with is some pretty immovable stuff, which really felt to me like it was on a cellular level...and that as good as the verbal therapy was that I had, and as much as I had cognitive insight about some of those patterns, they were still there.

And the idea of addressing that more directly through the brain, so that it wasn't consciousness-based, but that the treatment was really going straight to the fear, or to the "crazy" part – that seemed to make a lot of sense to me.

"So that's when I started with the neurofeedback. One of the things I wanted to find out was what I was doing when I was meditating. So I would hook myself up or I would have my partner hook me up to the neurofeedback machine, and I would just sit and sort of see what was going on with my brain when I was sitting and what brain wave states corresponded with...a certain kind of relaxed, alert, liberated state."

After a few experimental sessions using the neurofeedback equipment to assess her brain activity while meditating, Edie was able to set a protocol for her training. She set the "reward" at 8 - 11 hertz frequency, and then gradually raised the amplitudes.

"What I found," Edie relates, "was that if I practiced with focusing sensation in my entire body at once, the amplitude started to climb. And you can't think while you're focusing on sensation in your whole body, when you're really focusing on the sensations.

For me practicing meditation is about learning to stay with myself – to stay in sensation, to stay in the present, to stay out of complex thought."

Edie says that it's almost like having a 'meditation instructor inside my head'.

"You know, when you meditate without the neurofeedback machine," she says, "you could be spending half an hour planning dinner before you catch yourself. When you're hooked up to the neurofeedback machine, in two seconds you're getting feedback that you've gone off focus."

Edie was astounded at the energy level she experienced by combining neurofeedback with meditation.

"I've trained a bunch of times in just increasing the amplitude in high alpha, 11 hertz, and I didn't even know what that would feel like," she says, "so I decided to just try that. When I started the training, I think that the amplitude was at around 10 microvolts. Within two sessions, I could reliably go from 10 microvolts to 36 microvolts, which, as you know, is a huge increase. And what would happen is this feeling of huge amounts of energy...it was almost like I couldn't contain it."

Edie explains, "you are recruiting more and more neurons at that frequency."

The amazing energy level wasn't the only surprise Edie experienced while using the neurofeedback equipment during her meditation sessions. "Fairly reliably at about 32 microvolts," she says, "something would seem incredibly funny. I don't know what is being triggered in the brain. Sometimes there would be an image...a lot of the time, it was just a sense of how incredibly funny it was to be human."

Another benefit Edie experienced as a result of her combined meditation and neurotherapy sessions was improved sleep, in spite of having fibromyalgia. Like many fibromyalgia sufferers, Edie had not been producing enough low-wave brain activity to enter a deep sleep, but that has changed, and she now reports having much more restful sleep.

Summing up her experience, Edie says, "I think that meditation and neurofeedback training are very similar, and what the neurofeedback does is that it gives you very clear, objective concentration.

"All of the frequencies of the brain are always there, and it's not that any one frequency is good or better than another. For me the goal is to be able to selectively choose to use my brain in the way that's most appropriate for what I need to use my brain for in any given moment."

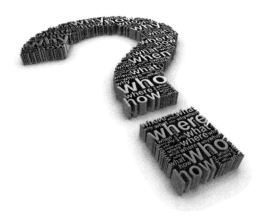

Commonly Asked Questions

What qualifications should I look for in a Neurofeedback clinician?

It is important to see the therapist or clinician you will be working with as an integral part of the outcome. It's tempting, considering the fact that studies have shown that neurofeedback does not rely on the placebo effect, to view the clinician as someone who is simply attaching the leads and calibrating the equipment, getting it ready for the session to begin. This would be a mistake.

Even with a tool and method of treatment as powerful and effective as neurofeedback, the relationship between the patient or client, and the therapist or clinician, remains one of the most important factors in the treatment outcome.

So, first and foremost, see how much you like, and feel comfortable with a therapist/clinician as the primary benchmark for selection. If you like them, proceed to the other factors such as their education level, years of experience, other methods of treatment they utilize, etc.; if you do not like them, STOP, and continue your search elsewhere.

Early in my career, while I was flattered by the number of people that expressed to me how warm, kind, considerate, etc. they found me to be, I was quick to discount these compliments as peripheral content, as far as what really mattered was concerned. Fortunately, I long ago realized that these aspects were the foundation for all else. Its importance is paramount.

How many sessions will I need?

While I'd love to be able to say something as specific and reassuring as "Sixty-two", I cannot. Yes, for many of the issues that someone may present, there is often an average number of treatments required, based on case studies and research results.

For the most part, these numbers are a good place to start, in terms of what you can expect as far as the number of treatments or sessions required. And, having said that, realize that for you, or a loved one, it may end up being more, or it may be that you achieve the results you are looking for with fewer sessions than the average number would suggest.

An example of an average number of sessions would be 40 for ADD, while other issues may be resolved in only 20, and still others may take 60 or more.

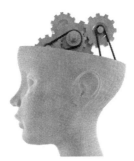

How does each neurofeedback session begin?

With most neurofeedback sessions, leads (thin wires sometimes called electrodes) are lightly pressed to the scalp by using a small amount of a conducting gel. These leads are allowing the electricity *from* your brain to travel to a computer that will quickly process this information, and translate it into what you will see on the screen in front of you.

Where are the sessions conducted?

Because of the compact size of the equipment used for neurofeedback, the sessions can be conducted just about anywhere you could put a computer and a couple of chairs. The most likely location will be in an office setting, much like you would expect if you were going to see a therapist, counselor or other healthcare provider.

Are there any side effects?

It's extremely rare for someone to experience side effects, and fortunately, any that might be experienced are short term, and usually disappear in less than 48 hours. The most common side effects are described as being "wired, tired, or irritated" During the session, your brain is working, putting out effort as it begins to self-regulate. You may feel like taking a nap, or you may feel like going for a walk. Just remember, most people will experience nothing they can distinguish or would classify as a side effect"

Should I do neurofeedback sessions if I'm pregnant?

There are few contraindications to using neurofeedback. In most cases, there would be no known reason to not engage in neurofeedback if you are pregnant. Please consult your physician before beginning to make sure you have all the bases covered.

Do I have to stop taking my medication while doing the neurofeedback treatment?

You should never stop taking your medication unless you have consulted with your physician. In most cases, taking medication while being treated with neurofeedback will not prevent a successful treatment.

How old do children have to be before they can receive neurofeedback treatment?

While there is no hard and fast rule or minimum age, children as young as 5 years of age have benefitted from neurofeedback. While treating children younger than 5 is not common, it's not necessarily unfeasible, either. This can best be determined by visiting with a neurofeedback therapist or clinician.

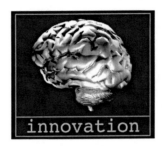

How was neurofeedback discovered?

Believe it, or not, it all started with cats. It was discovered that when cats were trained with specific frequencies, toxic chemicals that were known to cause seizures in cats could be blocked from their normal convulsive effects. It was later found that the same result could be achieved in both monkeys and humans.

Why haven't I heard more about neurofeedback from my Doctor or other healthcare providers?

First, realize there's no conspiracy. There are simply the "self-interest" and "awareness" factors at work. Let's look at the self-interest factor first. If you earn a living mowing lawns, for example, you probably wouldn't go out of your way to tell people about a new invention that can be poured on their lawn to put their grass in a sort of permanent, lush-green hibernation, allowing them to never have to mow again. This wouldn't make you a bad person; you are not required to put yourself out of business.

Then, we have the awareness (or lack thereof) factor. Most healthcare providers are very busy. It can be challenging just to stay current with all of the changes in their field that deal with what they *already* know and work with. It's quite possible that your current health care providers simply are not all that familiar with how quickly neurofeedback has evolved, and of the mounting research that continues to suggest that it should be considered for many different problems.

My neighbor say's that neurofeedback is nothing more than the placebo effect. Is that true?

Your neighbor means well. The voice they are speaking with is one of fear, and misunderstanding. First, it's highly unlikely that they know anything about neurofeedback, the principles involved, and the research available that clearly demonstrates its effectiveness.

Next, "the placebo effect", while being a term that's commonly tossed about by people from virtually all levels of education and profession, is largely misunderstood. Animals do not respond to a placebo; keep in mind, neurofeedback originated with the results that were achieved with cats.

A very revealing question, when asked with the appropriate attitude, is to simply respond to your neighbors claims with "Interesting, how do you know this?" When this question is asked, both you and your neighbor will rapidly discover that they really didn't gather any quality information regarding their position, and when it is all said and done, they were simply telling you their opinion, about what they thought the truth was concerning neurofeedback.

Remember, they most likely mean well, but as you know, people often initially resist the things they don't understand.

How long do the results last?

The results tend to be long term. I'm hesitant to say permanent but there is nothing at this point to discount this possibility for some people. After 40 sessions for ADHD, for example, the results usually last far into the future, and prove very resistant to fading.

How often do I need to have a neurofeedback session?

Sessions may be as few as 1 per week, or as often as 5 times a week. On average, most clinicians will suggest 2-3 sessions per week.

Are other forms of treatment ever used in conjunction with neurofeedback?

Neurofeedback may at times be used as a standalone treatment. However, some conditions benefit from incorporating neurofeedback with other methods of treatment such as cognitive therapy, hypnosis, or EMDR, for example. I prefer to view neurofeedback as a relatively new tool in my tool box that does not requires me to throw all of my other tools away, to be able to use it.

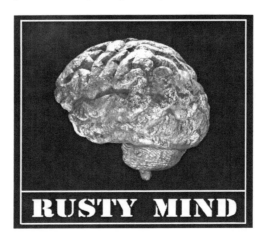

Does something have to be "wrong" with me to be able to benefit from neurofeedback?

No! There are times when someone may tear out perfectly good carpet from their home, simply because they want to install an *even better* grade or style of carpet. In this same way, many already high performing and functioning people, choose to use neurofeedback to fine tune their brain, allowing it to function in an *even more refined* and polished manner.

What's the future of neurofeedback?

The most recent research on neurofeedback is very exciting and compelling, making it very hard for even most skeptical and resistant people to ignore. As the awareness of neurofeedback grows, it will become more and more mainstream, and be used by more and more health care providers, until one day, it is as common a treatment as aspirin.

Do I need to do anything special to prepare for my neurofeedback session?

Not really. Some things that may help, however, include:

- Showing up well rested.
- Have your scalp relatively clean so a good connection can be made with the leads.

- Have something to eat (preferably high in protein) an h(
  before your session.
- Be willing to relax during the session without "trying" to make
  things happen. "Trying" implies effort, and this will interfere with
  the process.

Case Study – From Traumatic Brain Injury – to Peace and Bliss – Debi Dusold

I suffered a traumatic brain injury ten years ago in an auto accident.

I spent 5 years with severe deficits in memory, attention, organizing, balance, headaches, and uncharacteristic emotional outbursts.

I was unable to work for two years.

I could not keep seven digits in my head so dialing a phone number was a major undertaking.

Did my shoes go on first or my socks?

I had to learn to never, ever leave the kitchen if I had turned on a gas burner.

I was told by my primary care doctor, a neurologist, a chiropractor, a physical therapist, and a neuropsychologist that there was nothing I could do but learn to cope.

When a psychologist told me that my memory loss could be due to "getting to be that age" I finally got mad enough to look outside of the mainstream medical arena for help.

Through a fluke, I finally found neurofeedback and within 25 sessions I was pretty much back to normal.

I got inspired by my own healing experience and started a business called 'MindWorks Studio' in Tucson, Arizona.

Since I had access to lots of different equipment, I kept on doing neurofeedback on myself. I kept getting better in ways I had not anticipated.

Eventually my usual state became one of peace, joy, tranquility, and equanimity.

I was a very unhappy, depressed, driven person even before brain injury.

About six months ago it became apparent that something strange was going on. I could not interact with friends and family the same way I always had before. I began experiencing some very unusual states of consciousness.

It was difficult to believe that no one else felt happy, peaceful, stress free and loving ALL THE TIME like I do.

Nothing fazes me. No fear. No anxiety. No hatred or ill will towards anyone.

I started meditating without any instruction and found it to be effortless.

This bliss just never goes away. It's been about two years now.

I finally sought out a Buddhist meditation master who interviewed me at length. His analysis was that I was exhibiting the preliminary stages of enlightenment. Who ME?!

Together we have formed an organization called The 'Parallel Paths Institute' to study how neurofeedback can rapidly accelerate the goals of meditation.

I think that if I can do this anyone can.

Neurofeedback can go way beyond just healing from neurological problems.

It keeps on getting better.

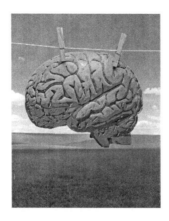

Closing Thoughts

It's amazing to consider that not that long ago physicians thought of hand washing as an unnecessary inconvenience. As a result men, women and children died from simple infections that could have easily been prevented had they only known about microbes.

Neurofeedback Tip

It's amazing to consider that it's not been all that long ago, that physicians thought of hand washing as an unnecessary inconvenience. As a result men, women and children died from simple infections that could have easily been prevented had they have only known about microbes.

Because they could not see microbes, believing in their existence defied the logic of the day. Then, in one fell swoop, the microscope changed everything; once doctors could actually see the wiggling organisms, on a thin glass plate beneath them, the idea of washing their hands before surgery suddenly made sense. Seeing, in this case, was believing.

Neurofeedback Tip

Neurofeedback is the epitome of "seeing is believing" To actually be able to see what the brain is doing, in real time, and continue to watch as it changes makes improvements, shifting effortlessly form one frequency to another, depending on the context and the task at hand, is nothing short of a beautiful display of the complexity of the human brain and nervous system.

Neurofeedback is the epitome of "seeing is believing." Actually being able to see what the brain is doing, in real time, and continue to watch as it changes and makes improvements, shifting effortlessly from one frequency to another (depending on the context and the task at hand) is nothing short of a beautiful display of the complexity of the human brain and nervous system.

While I can't know the exact reason(s) why you picked up this book, I can assume that either you or a loved one - or both - have been dealing with some type of challenge that you've found to be interfering with some aspect of your life.

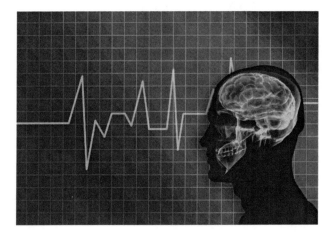

Neurofeedback is changing lives. Never before have we been able to so adequately and precisely work with the human brain to bring about the exciting changes, that so many others were able to enjoy. Will you be next?

If you find yourself wondering just how quickly and profoundly you will be able to experience the delight of a different life, let that be an indication that what you have been wondering about is a very real possibility.

If you consider your current challenges, what will it cost you, in terms of your quality of life, if you were still dealing with this issue 1 year, 5 years, or even 10 years from now? As it turns out, some of the things people have been told, such as *"you'll just have to learn to live with it"*, are no longer true; we have seen evidence that indicates otherwise for several conditions.

Now, if your life were to change significantly, in terms of the "problem" you wish to resolve, and were to do so within the next 6 months, how much more enjoyment would you get out of life? How many more opportunities could you take part in with your family, friends and loved ones?

I trust that you can already think about certain sections of this book that have made you stop and say "Ah ha!" and have caused you to catch a glimpse of alternative outcomes that you may have at one time written off as unlikely. As you find your curiosity deepening, and your willingness to explore the use of neurofeedback growing, know that I share your excitement, and would consider it an honor (as I'm sure many clinicians would) to assist on your journey towards a more pleasant and enjoyable way of living. I hope to meet you one day...be well!

Bibliography

Demos, John, M. "Getting Started with Neurofeedback" New York: W.W. Norton & Co., 2004.

Dustman, Robert E. 1990. Age and Fitness Effects of EEG, ERP's, Visual Sensitivity and Cognition. *Neurobiology of Aging*. Vol. 11(3), 193.

Fehmi, Les., and Robbins, Jim "The Open Focus Brain: Harnessing the Power of Attention to Heal Mind and Body." New York: Trumpeter, 2008.

Green, Elmer, and Alyce Green. "Biofeedback and States of Consciousness." In *Handbook of States of Consciousness*. New York: Van Nostrand Reinhold, 1986.

Larsen, Stephen. "The Healing Power of Neurofeedback: The Revolutionary LENS Technique for Restoring Optimal Brain Function." Vermont: Healing Arts Press, 2006.

Linden, M., T. Habib, and V. Tadojevic. "A Controlled Study of the Effects of EEG Biofeedback on the Cognition and Behavior of Children with Attention Deficit Disorders and Leraning Disabilities." *Biofeedback and Self Regulation* 21, no. 1 (1996): 35-49.

Lubar, J.F.; Swartwood, M.O.; Swartwood, J.N.; O'Donnell, P.H. (1995). "Evaluation of the Effectiveness of EEG Neurofeedback Training for ADHD in a Clinical Setting as Measured by Changes in TOVA Scores, Behavioral Ratings, and WISC-R Performance". *Applied Psychophysiology and Biofeedback* **20** (1): 83–99.

Mueller, H., S. Donaldson, D. Nelson, and M. Layman. "Treatment of Fibromyalgia Incorporating EEG –Driven Stimulation: A Clinical Outcomes Study." *Journal of Clinical Psychology*, 57, no. 7 (2001): 933-52.

Othmer, Siegfried F., Susan Othmer, and Clifford S. Marks. "EEG Biofeedback Training for ADD, Specific Learning Disabilities and Associated Conduct Problems." *EEG Spectrum*, September 1991.

Peniston, E. "EEG Alpha-Theta Neurofeedback: Promising Clinical Approach for Future Psychotherapy and Medicine." *Megabrain Report: The Journal of Mind Technology* 2, no. 4 (1994): 40-43.

Pert, Candace. Molecules of Emotion, New York, NY: Scribner, 1997.

Robbins, Jim. "A Symphony in the Brain: The Evolution of the New Brain Wave Biofeedback." New York: Grove Press, 2008.

Sapolsky, Robert, M. "Why Zebras Don't Get Ulcers: The Acclaimed Guide to Stress, Stress-Related Diseases, and Coping." New York: Owl Books, 2004.

Steinberg, Mark, and Othmer, Sigfried. "ADD: The 20 Hour Solution. Oregon: Robert Reed Publishers, 2004.

Siebert, Al. "The Resiliency Advantage: Master Change, Thrive Under Pressure, and Bounce BCK from Setbacks." San Francisco: Berrett Koehler, 2005.

Sterman, M.B. "Studies of EEG Biofeedback Training in Men and Cats." *In Highlights of 17ᵗʰ Annual Conference: VA Cooperative Studies in Mental Health and Behavioral Sciences,* vol. PP.5060. Veterans' Administration, 1972.

Swindle, Paul, G. "Neurofeedback: How Neurotherapy Effectively Treats Depression, ADHD, Autism, and More." North Carolina: Rutgers University Press, 2008.

About the Author

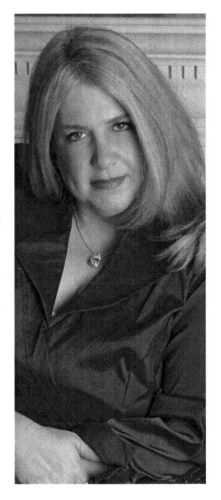

Dr. Clare Albright is a Clinical Psychologist and neurofeedback provider in Lake Forest, CA.

She has been counseling in Orange County, CA for over 25 years, and is the proud mother of an 11 year old son.

Dr. Albright has been a public speaker for over three decades and is available to speak with your group about

- neurofeedback,
- peak performance
- parenting
- staying close to your child
- positive child discipline
- parenting adolescents
- ADHD and ADD
- anxiety disorders
- autism
- Asperger's Disorder
- training counselors
- etc.

Dr. Albright will 'wow' your group with her warm, humorous, educational, and inspiring presentation.

Dr. Albright is a graduate of Coach University and provides life coaching services by telephone and by Skype all over the globe.

Dr. Albright can be reached at (949) 454-0996.

Breinigsville, PA USA
27 September 2010
246182BV00004B/3/P